The 5-Ingredient LOW-CARB DIET Cookbook

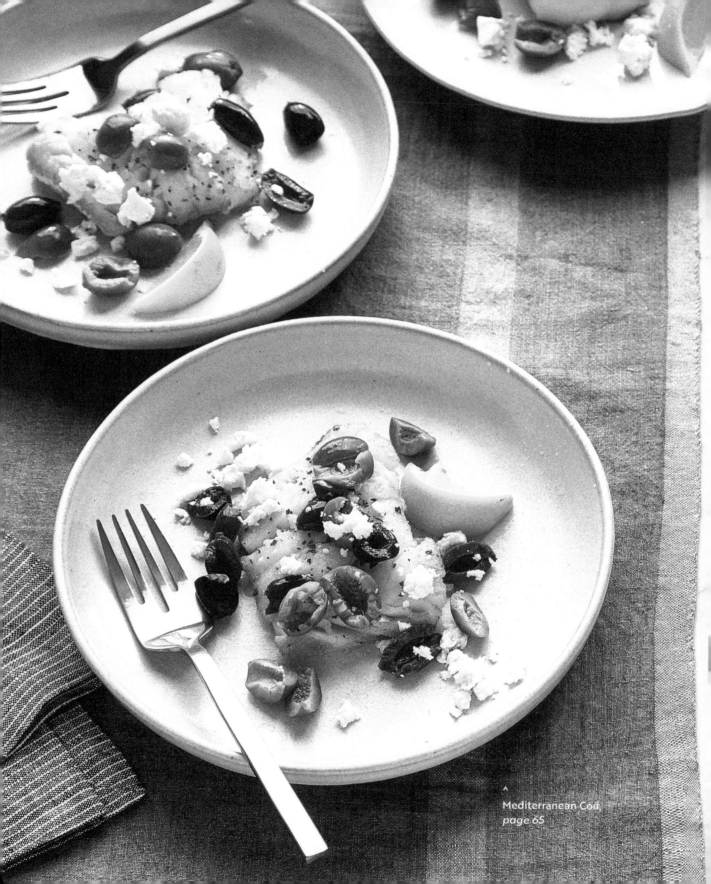

Mediterranean Cod,
page 65

Bek Davis   PHOTOGRAPHY BY **Hélène Dujardin**

The 5-Ingredient
LOW-CARB DIET
Cookbook

100 Easy Recipes for
Better Health

ROCKRIDGE
PRESS

For general information on our other products and services or to obtain technical support, please contact our Customer Care Department within the United States at (866) 744-2665, or outside the United States at (510) 253-0500.

Rockridge Press publishes its books in a variety of electronic and print formats. Some content that appears in print may not be available in electronic books, and vice versa.

TRADEMARKS: Rockridge Press and the Rockridge Press logo are trademarks or registered trademarks of Callisto Media Inc. and/or its affiliates, in the United States and other countries, and may not be used without written permission. All other trademarks are the property of their respective owners. Rockridge Press is not associated with any product or vendor mentioned in this book.

Interior & Cover Designer: Jay Dea
Art Producer: Janice Ackerman
Editor: Adrian Potts
Production Editor: Matt Burnett

Photography: © 2019 Helen Dujardin.
Food styled by Anna Hampton

ISBN: Print 978-1-64611-524-2
eBook 978-1-64611-525-9
R0

In loving memory of my amazing Ma, who taught me that food should always be enjoyed.

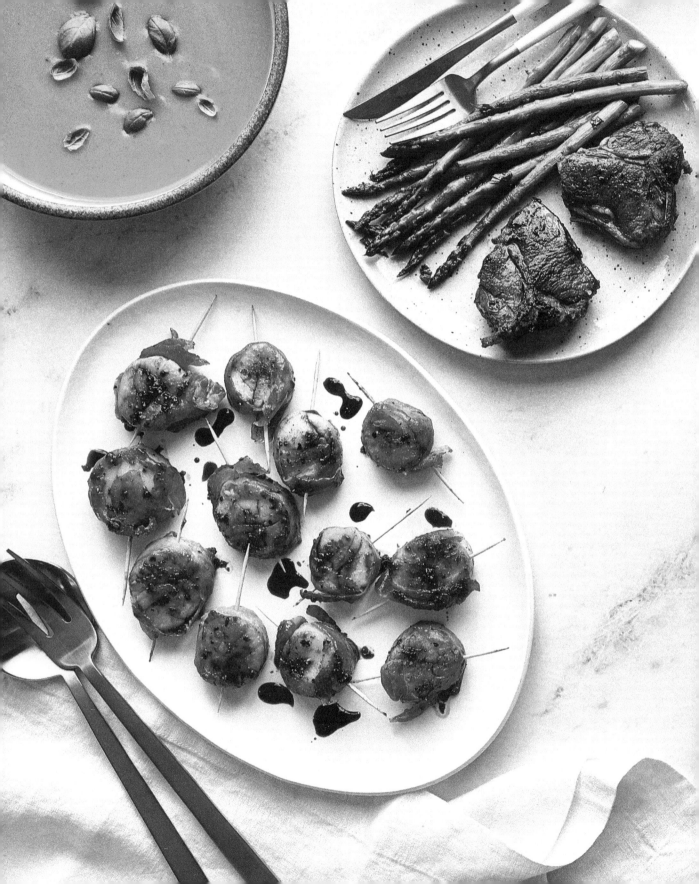

Contents

< Prosciutto-Wrapped Sea Scallops with Balsamic Glaze, *page 58* • Red Pepper Soup, *page 30*
Lamb Chops with Lemon-and-Mint Asparagus, *page 92*

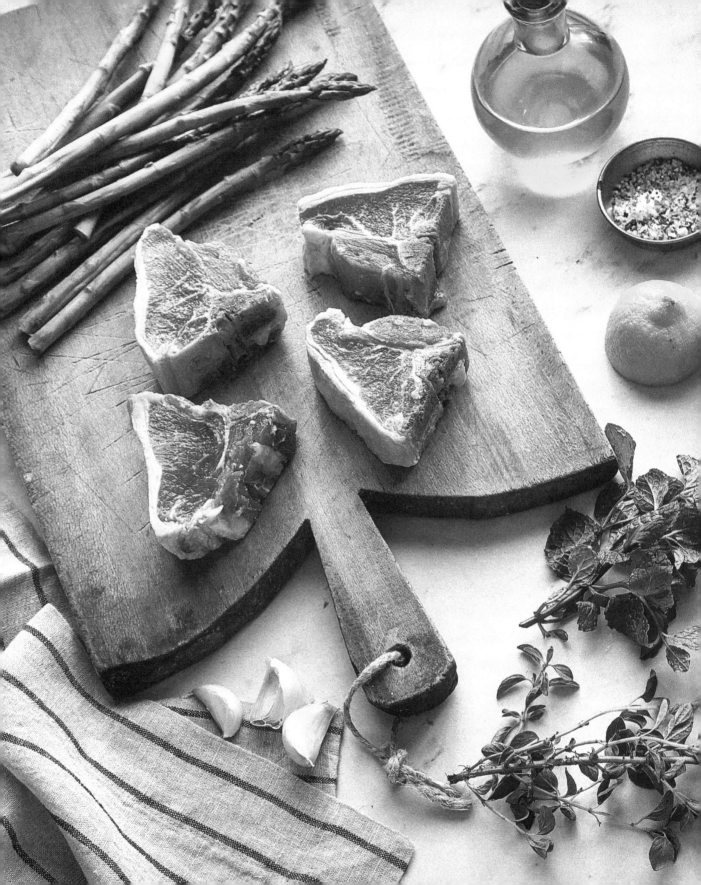

Introduction

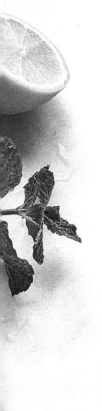

I come from a large foodie family where the kitchen was the nucleus of the home. Our kitchen was always "open for business," and together we dreamed up, tried out, and successfully created many recipes. Unsurprisingly, cooking became one of my greatest passions, which I went on to formalize as a graduate of Culinary Arts Institute of Louisiana.

Unfortunately, I allowed my passion to take over my waistline. Following the birth of my second child, I found myself staring at a scale reading almost 200 pounds. At this weight, I needed to be at least seven feet tall for a normal BMI; at five feet tall, I can barely ride the rides at an amusement park! I was miserable, physically and mentally. Diabetes runs in my family, so I knew I needed to drop the excess weight and get healthy. Knowing this lit a fire within me, and, after some careful research, I decided to try low-carb eating.

Within weeks of adopting a low-carb diet, my weight began to decrease, my joints stopped aching, and my skin looked healthier. Before long, I was jumping out of bed each morning with an abundance of energy and finding it much easier to move around without becoming winded.

I know there are many reasons why cooking nutritious food at home can seem like a challenge; lack of time and the energy to cook are usually the main culprits. After a long and busy day, it's all too easy to grab a carb-loaded meal from the freezer aisle of a supermarket or a local fast food drive-thru.

But cooking low-carb doesn't have to mean sacrificing time or taste. As the recipes in this book will show, using a small number of familiar and fresh ingredients will not only save time at the grocery store and in the kitchen, but it will also save you money—all while creating flavorful, low-carb meals that are sure to please any crowd and set you on a path to better health.

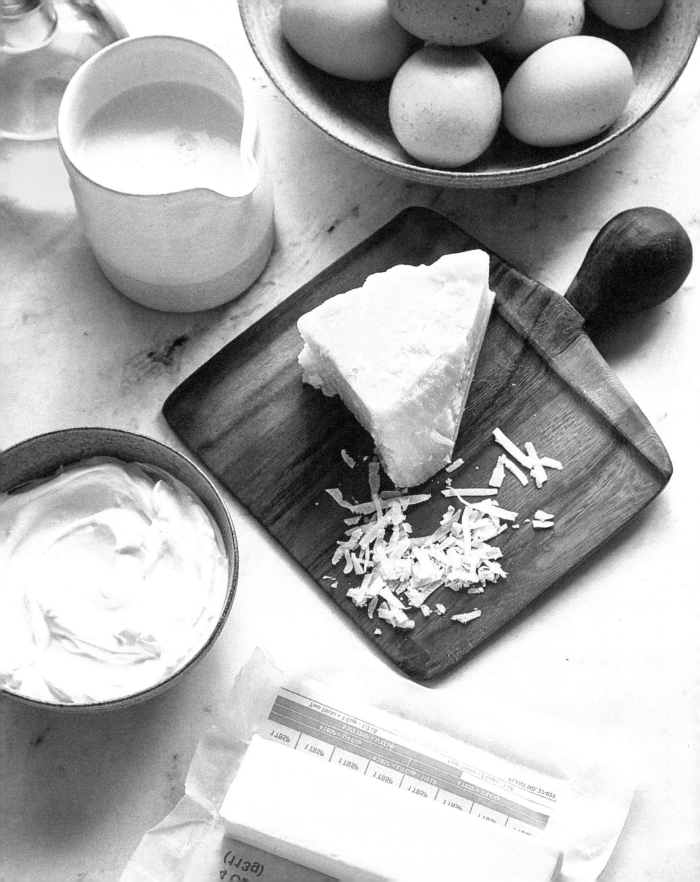

1.

Easy Low-Carb Cooking

Over the past five years, I have found that a low-carb diet makes sense and is very sustainable. Just like with any task, in order to be successful, you need the know-how and proper tools if you want to achieve your goals. I will show you that a low-carb diet is not complicated, and together we will put the fun back into cooking delicious, healthy, low-carb meals using just a few familiar and affordable ingredients. Food is meant to be enjoyed and should never be a source of stress. As I learned in the culinary world, the best dishes always use simple ingredients and are cooked simply. In this chapter, I'll explain the basics of what you'll need to start your low-carb journey.

Low-Carb Eating

In today's busy world, there is so much noise out there about diets. As a lifetime diet junkie, I know it can be quite overwhelming to find the diet that works best for your body, and I share the frustration of trying to determine how best to start. You are not alone; this was my struggle for many decades. Since I didn't have a blueprint for all of those years, I ended up experimenting with many fad diets until finding success with the low-carb diet.

What is the Low-Carb Diet?

A low-carb diet deliberately limits starchy carbohydrates and focuses on proteins, healthy fats, and low-carb fruits and vegetables. While many people follow a low-carb diet for weight loss, which may be your main motivating factor, a diet that avoids simple carbohydrates is also recommended to help reverse prediabetes and treat type 2 diabetes.

Carbohydrates are one of the three macronutrients, along with fat and protein, that your body requires to survive on a daily basis. Carbs are the main source of food that your body uses for energy. After consuming carbs, your body converts them into glucose (blood sugar), which is used to give your body the necessary energy to function. Carbs fall into two vastly different categories: simple and complex.

Simple carbohydrates can be found in refined sugar, corn syrup and high-fructose corn syrup, fruit juices, sodas, candy, and processed foods. They have a simple chemical structure, and because of this, your body quickly uses these carbohydrates for energy. As a result, you will often experience a rise in blood sugar when you eat them. Simple carbs offer very little or no nutritional value for your body.

Complex carbohydrates, on the other hand, can be found in whole grains, nuts, beans, fruits, and vegetables. As the name suggests, they have a more complex chemical structure. Many of these carbs provide your body with needed vitamins, minerals, and fiber. The complexity of these carbs results in a longer digestion time, which in turn has less of an impact on your blood sugar. The majority of your carbs should come from complex carbohydrates.

According to the Mayo Clinic, a daily limit of 20 to 60 grams (0.7 to 2 ounces) of carbs per day is typical for a low-carb diet for weight loss. These amounts will provide 80 to 240 calories.

Those taking a more moderate approach—perhaps seeking steady weight loss or to maintain a healthy weight—might choose to consume more than this amount, with the upper range of the diet falling around 150 grams of net carbs per day (net carbs equal the total carbs minus the fiber). However, your body is unique and your daily intake may need to be altered to get the results you are seeking.

The Health Benefits

Many come to the low-carb diet to address a particular health issue.

Weight loss: On a basic level, restricting carbs forces your body to burn its fat stores for energy. Replacing simple carbs from processed foods with protein, fat, and complex carbs will also leave you feeling less hungry. Healthy fats and lean proteins help the body stay full longer. While fibrous carbs—such as spinach, kale, celery, and broccoli—take longer to break down than their simple-carb counterparts, they also help keep hunger at bay and reduce your calorie intake.

Reduce heart disease: According to research by the Harvard School of Public Health, a moderately low-carb diet can help reduce heart disease, as long as protein and fat selections come from healthy sources.

Lower risk for type 2 diabetes: Harvard research also found that a similarly low-carb diet with healthy protein and fat sources is also effective in combating prediabetes and preventing its progression to diabetes.

Reduce blood sugar: Consuming fewer carbs can also help those with diabetes better manage their blood sugar levels. Carbs raise blood glucose more than other foods, so the body must produce more insulin to digest them. While this is particularly true for simple carbs, many complex carbs have a low glycemic index. The index, which ranges from 0 to 100, measures how quickly a type of carb raises blood sugar. The lower the number, the slower blood-sugar levels are raised.

Lower cholesterol: According to the Mayo Clinic, low-carb diets may improve high-density lipoprotein (HDL) cholesterol and triglyceride values slightly more than moderate-carb diets. In other words, they can help lower cholesterol and improve your heart health. That may be due not only to how many carbs you eat but also to the quality of your other food choices. Lean protein (fish, poultry, and legumes), healthy fats (monounsaturated and polyunsaturated), and unprocessed carbs (whole grains, legumes, vegetables, fruits, and low-fat dairy products) are generally better choices.

A LOW-CARB LIFESTYLE CHANGE

When done properly, a low-carb diet is filled with many nutritious and delicious foods. The goal is not to eliminate all carbs—the human body needs them to function after all—but rather to consume healthy carbs in combination with other wholesome foods. Instead of viewing this as a fad diet, look at it as part of a long-term lifestyle change that is 100 percent sustainable.

Of course, as with any health issues and dietary changes, it is best to consult your physician first to consider your particular circumstances and goals.

The Low-Carb Diets

There are a number of more specific low-carb diets, some of which target rapid weight loss. However, many find that a more moderate (i.e., less restrictive) intake of carbs can be more sustainable for the long-term. While the recipes in this book cater to a moderate range of carbs, many will be suitable for different diet types.

Keto: The keto diet is a low-carb, high-fat diet (LCHF) that aims to put your body into a state of ketosis in which your body is deprived of its normal quick energy source (glucose from carbs) and burns fat instead. The macro ratios on the keto diet are very strict: 70 percent fat, 25 percent protein, 5 percent carbs, with a typical intake of 20 to 50 grams net carbs per day. However, most people following this diet stay around 20 grams net carbs.

Paleo: This is a low-carb diet that focuses on whole foods that were obtained by hunting, fishing, and gathering during the Paleolithic Period. Foods typically include lean meats, fish, vegetables, fruits, nuts, and seeds. The Paleo diet eliminates refined foods, dairy, and sweeteners. The carb intake ranges from 50 to 150 grams due to the inclusion of starchy roots, fruits, and vegetables in this diet.

Atkins: Like keto, the goal of the Atkins diet is to force your body into a state of ketosis to burn fat. Atkins offers three low-carb diet plans based upon your dietary needs and goals. The carb intake options on Atkins are 20, 40, and 100 grams net carbs.

Getting Started

When I decided to take control of my health and adapt to a low-carb diet, my first priority was to set an official "start date" and to take steps to set myself up for success. I removed all processed and carb-loaded foods from my kitchen and followed up with a trip to the supermarket to fill my pantry and refrigerator with healthy low-carb foods. I started off with basics. I kept my meals very simple with limited ingredients. Every meal would consist of a protein, two cups of low-carb vegetables, and a serving of a healthy fat. Simplifying my meals made for an easier transition while I was learning a new eating lifestyle, and it also helped create a new (healthy) habit; it can do all of this for you, too.

How will I feel to begin with?

Your body will go through changes when transitioning to a low-carb diet. You may get headaches due to the lack of sugar and carbs. This is why it's important to increase your salt and water intake to keep your electrolytes and hydration in check. You may initially find that your energy level is lower than you're used to and that you become tired more easily than usual, but this soon will pass. Cravings are also common. If you crave carbs, create a distraction. Go for a walk, do laundry, or clean your house. It takes a few weeks to form a habit. You've got this!

Will I eat more proteins and fats?

The overall approach for the recipes in this book is low-carb, moderate protein, and healthy fats. When adopting a low-carb diet, you are limiting your carb intake. Therefore, you will be replacing those calories with an increase of proteins and healthy fats.

It is not necessary to overindulge in proteins. If you consume too much protein, your body won't be able to break it down, and it will be forced to convert the proteins into sugar, which you want to avoid.

Despite their bad reputation, fats play an important role in any diet. Fat gives the body energy, supports cell growth, helps the body absorb nutrients, and gives you the feeling of being full and satisfied. The fats we use to fuel ourselves should always be nutritious, healthy fats that benefit the body. Some of the fats you will see frequently in the recipes are avocados, nuts, whole eggs, extra-virgin olive oil, and fatty fish.

Tips for Success

I encourage you to keep a food diary. Using a nutrition counter is also very helpful when starting a new diet. There are many free apps and websites that are available to simplify this process. Seeing what you eat on a daily basis will keep you motivated and serve as a useful resource when needed.

Embrace the entire low-carb lifestyle by reading books and online publications about the low-carb diet. The more you educate yourself, the easier it becomes to stay on track and motivated.

Find your support tribe! Social media is a wonderful outlet for support. The low-carb community on Instagram and Facebook is large, extremely supportive, and very welcoming; this online community is a great resource and a motivational outlet for you as you travel along your low-carb journey.

Below is a list of foods for you to enjoy and limit while adapting a low-carb lifestyle. You will find that these lists are very helpful when menu-planning and shopping for groceries.

FOODS TO ENJOY

Dairy and Alternatives

- Almond milk (unsweetened)
- Cheese
- Coconut milk (unsweetened)
- Cream cheese
- Eggs
- Greek yogurt
- Half-and-half
- Heavy whipping cream
- Sour cream

Fats

- Avocado oil
- Butter
- Coconut butter
- Coconut oil
- Extra-virgin olive oil
- Ghee
- Grapeseed oil
- Macadamia oil
- Mayonnaise
- MCT oil
- Nut butters (no sugar added)
- Sesame oil

Flavor Enhancers

- Dried spices (no sugar)
- Herbs
- Lemon
- Lime

- Mustard (Dijon & yellow)
- Soy sauce

Fruits

- Avocados
- Blackberries
- Blueberries
- Cantaloupe
- Clementines
- Coconut
- Cranberries
- Kiwi
- Lemons
- Vinegar

- Limes
- Olives
- Peaches
- Pears
- Plums
- Raspberries
- Strawberries
- Tomatoes

Meats (Lean Cuts)

- Beef
- Chicken
- Lamb
- Pork
- Turkey

Nuts and Seeds

- Almonds
- Brazil nuts
- Cashews (in moderation)
- Chia seeds
- Flaxseed
- Hazelnuts
- Hemp seeds
- Macadamia nuts
- Peanuts
- Pecans
- Pine nuts
- Pistachios (in moderation)
- Pumpkin seeds
- Sesame seeds
- Walnuts

Seafood

- Fish
- Octopus
- Shellfish
- Squid

Vegetables

- Acorn and butternut squash (in moderation)
- Artichokes
- Asparagus
- Beets
- Broccoli
- Cabbage
- Carrots

- Cauliflower
- Celery
- Collard greens
- Cucumbers
- Eggplants
- Green beans
- Leafy greens (e.g., chard, kale, spinach)
- Mushrooms

- Onions
- Peas
- Peppers
- Pumpkin
- Sprouts
- Turnips
- Yellow squash
- Zucchini

FOODS TO LIMIT OR AVOID

Dairy and Alternatives

- Cow milk
- Nut milk (sweetened)
- Soy milk
- Yogurt

Grains

- Bread
- Oats
- Pasta
- Rice
- Wheat

Fruit

- Apples
- Bananas
- Cherries
- Dried fruit
- Pineapple
- Plantains

Vegetables

- Corn
- Potatoes
- Sweet Potatoes
- Yams

Meats and Alternatives

- Deli meats (with fillers and sugar)
- Sausage (with fillers and sugar)
- Seitan

Sweeteners

- High-fructose corn syrup
- Maple syrup
- Sugar (brown and white)

Prepare Your Kitchen

You don't have to be a master chef or have a restaurant-inspired kitchen to create the recipes in this book. However, there are some kitchen essentials that will make your life easier when preparing fresh, low-carb meals.

Essential Equipment

You probably already have most of the items on this list, but you will use these things to make many of the meals in this book. Following these are nice-to-have items, which will make cooking a little easier but are not required.

Baking Sheets: You will need at least one large baking sheet for your one-pan meals.

Blender: This will come in handy for making smoothies, sauces, dressings, and soups. Many companies sell combination blender/food processors that are fantastic.

Baking Dish: I recommend an 8-by-8-inch baking dish for smaller bakes and a 9-by-13-inch dish for larger ones.

Knives and Cutting Boards: It will be worth your while to invest in at least one chef's knife and one paring knife. You can find affordable, quality knives at most chain stores. For cutting boards, you will need one board for meats and another for fruits and vegetables. Many stores sell color-coded cutting boards for separate foods. I find these very useful for keeping a sanitary cooking environment.

Measuring Cups and Spoons: Measuring your ingredients on a low-carb diet is very important, especially if your goal is weight loss. The baked recipes in particular will require measuring to ensure they cook properly.

Mixing Bowls: You're going to be using mixing bowls more than you might expect. When meal prepping, I always have a mixing bowl on the counter for trash and food scraps. This saves me from having to run back and forth to the trash can and it keeps my work space tidy.

Nonstick Skillet: A 10-inch nonstick skillet will be needed for many of the recipes in this book.

Saucepan: A 3-quart saucepan should suffice for the recipes in this book.

Sauté Pan: A 10-inch sauté pan or skillet is the perfect size for most dishes.

Slow Cooker: There are a handful of recipes that require a slow cooker. This is your ultimate timesaver—throw in the ingredients, set the timer, and walk away.

Nice-to-Have Equipment

Cast Iron Skillet: My favorite skillet is a cast iron skillet because it is so versatile. It's great for egg bakes and quickly cooking foods at high temperatures. I would suggest at least a 10-inch cast iron skillet.

Cooling Racks: These racks are nice to have for cooling baked desserts.

Food Processor: I use a food processor in many recipes to cut down on prep time.

Immersion Blender: If you don't want to pull a big blender out, an immersion blender is what you need. You can easily blend soups, sauces, smoothies, and dressings without the hassle or time-consuming cleanup.

The Pantry Staples

There are a few basic staple ingredients you should have on hand to make the recipes in this book. They will appear in most of the recipes and do not count as part of the five main ingredients in each recipe, as they are considered general kitchen supplies that everyone should have. Make sure you have:

- Extra-virgin olive oil
- Freshly ground black pepper
- Garlic
- Lemons
- Salt

Low-Carb Cooking

Don't let cooking low-carb meals intimidate you. Because we are only working with five main ingredients and a handful of staple ingredients, you will spend less time in the grocery store and less time cooking. The recipes in this book are going to show you the basics of low-carb cooking that will set the foundation to help you create future meals.

Shopping Tips

I love grocery shopping; it's one of my favorite pastimes. When you are shopping, the majority of your time should be spent along the perimeter of the store. This is where you will find the fresh fruits, vegetables, dairy, and proteins. I like to call these "clean foods." The middle aisles tend to be filled with foods that are highly processed and carb- and sugar-loaded. Frozen vegetables, canned beans, canned tomatoes, and some canned vegetables are the exception. Frozen vegetables are extremely convenient, and I always keep some of those on hand.

Products being promoted as "low-fat" can be filled with hidden carbs. To maintain flavor, companies replace the fat in these products with sugars. Cow milk is another item with hidden carbs. Milk contains lactose, which is the natural sugar in dairy products. One cup of milk has about 12 grams of sugar. Surprisingly, bullions and broth powders are not just loaded with sugar but also cane sugars.

When reading food labels, look for simplicity. The ingredient list should be minimal without sugars, fillers, or words you cannot pronounce. The fewer the ingredients, the healthier the product.

Clear Out High-Carb Items

It is time to remove the products that might be a temptation for you while transitioning to a low-carb lifestyle. Gather all sugar- and carb-loaded foods up and give them away. I am sure many friends and family members will happily take these foods off your hands. You may even consider donating the food to a homeless shelter or a nonprofit establishment.

Flavor Boosters

Cooking wholesome, low-carb dishes does not translate into flavorless meals. There are many fresh herbs and seasonings readily available that will bring your easy low-carb meals to the next level of flavor. Plant a small herb garden in a pot and place it in your kitchen window. Searing and roasting enhances the flavor profile of food by caramelizing and bringing out natural flavors. A simple squeeze of fresh citrus juice will brighten up a simple dish and make your taste buds dance. Don't hesitate to experiment with your food!

What About Sugar?

There are many food products stocked in American supermarkets that are processed and loaded with sugar. Avoiding foods that are high in sugar will greatly benefit your body. You may lose weight, have more energy, control diabetes, or prevent obesity. The human body does not need this added sugar to function.

In my recipes, you will find that I use natural sweeteners. These sweeteners have a low glycemic rating and do not raise blood sugar levels. My preference is for Swerve (erythritol), which is available in granulated, brown, and confectioners' varieties.

About the Recipes

The 100 recipes in this book are rooted in simplicity with delicious and bold flavors, using ingredients you can find in most grocery stores. Each dish calls for five main ingredients and a few staple pantry items mentioned earlier (olive oil, salt, pepper, garlic, and lemon) that do not count towards the main ingredients. For ease of reference, the five primary ingredients in each recipe have been highlighted in green.

You will also find the following labels that will assist you in planning your meals:

- 30-minute: The recipe can be prepped, cooked, and served in 30 minutes or less.
- Dairy-free: The recipe does not contain dairy.
- Gluten-free: The recipe does not contain gluten products.
- One-pot or pan: The recipe can be created using a single pot, pan, or sheet.
- Vegan: The recipe does not contain any meat, dairy, or animal products.
- Vegetarian: The recipe does not contain meat products.

At least half of the recipes in this book can either be made in a single pot or pan, or they can be prepped and cooked in 30 minutes or less.

Many of the recipes will also include the following tips:

- Ingredient tip: Ingredient suggestions, such as how to best select ingredients or prepare them more easily.
- Make it vegan/vegetarian: Suggestions for replacing animal products with vegetarian or vegan options.
- Simplify it: Time-saving or energy-saving tips to make the recipe more convenient.
- Substitution tip: Suggestions for replacing a less common ingredient with a more common one.
- Variation: Suggestions for adding or changing ingredients to mix things up a little or try something new with the recipe.

The recipes in this book are designed to serve four people. Increase or decrease the servings based upon your needs. Each recipe will have nutritional breakdowns, including total carbs and net carbs, listed per serving at the end of the recipe. The net carbs represent the total amount of carbs minus fiber. For example, total carbs (15g) − fiber (10g) = 5g net carbs.

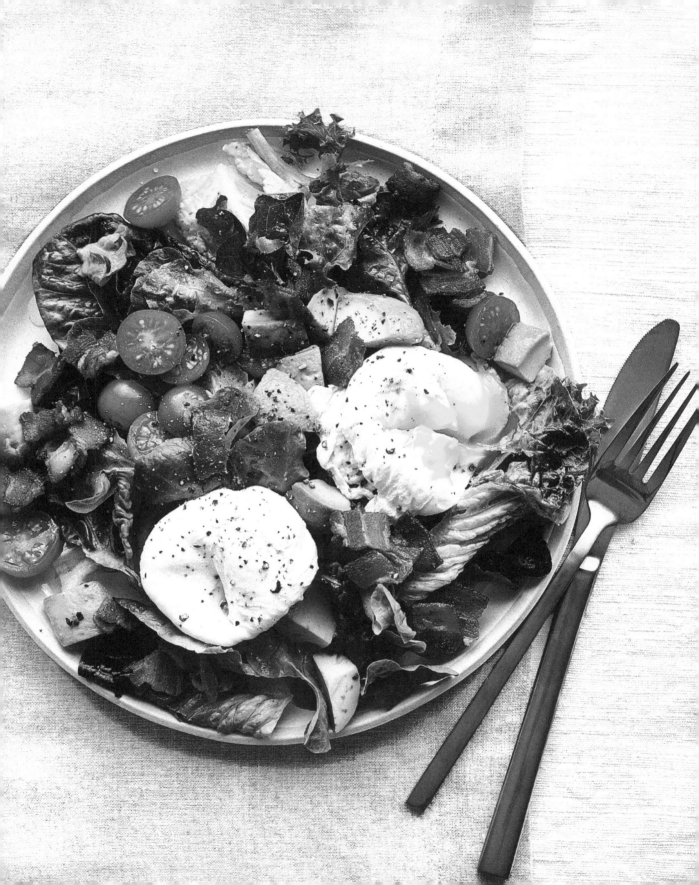

2.

Smoothies and Breakfasts

< Cobb Salad with Poached Eggs, *page 21*

Peanut Butter Smoothie

SERVES

PREP
TIME

Drinking this deliciously sweet low-carb smoothie is like having dessert for breakfast. The richness from the cocoa and peanut butter is quite decadent. When time is of the essence, this is the perfect on-the-go start to your morning.

¼ cup unsweetened cocoa powder

⅓ cup natural sugar-free peanut butter

2 cups unsweetened almond milk

4 teaspoons Swerve granulated sweetener

1 cup heavy whipping cream

½ teaspoon salt

Ice, as needed

1. In a blender, blend the cocoa powder, peanut butter, almond milk, Swerve, heavy whipping cream, and salt until smooth.

2. Add the ice, a couple of cubes at a time, and blend again until your desired consistency is reached.

Make it vegan: **Replace the heavy whipping cream with coconut cream. To add some extra nutrients, use frozen raspberries instead of ice to reach your desired consistency.**

Per Serving: **Calories: 413; Total Fat: 37g; Protein: 10g; Total Carbohydrates: 10g; Fiber: 4g; Net Carbs: 6g; Sweetener Carbs: 4g**

Macros: **Fat: 80%; Protein: 10%; Carbs: 10%**

Pumpkin and Cashew Smoothie

30-MINUTE / DAIRY-FREE / GLUTEN-FREE / VEGAN

There's no need to wait for pumpkin season to enjoy this protein-packed smoothie. The combination of protein from the cashews and high fiber from the pumpkin is sure to keep you going throughout your morning.

4 cups unsweetened almond milk or another nut milk

1 cup canned pure pumpkin purée

1 cup unsalted cashews

3 teaspoons Swerve granulated sweetener

2 teaspoons pumpkin pie spice

½ teaspoon salt

Ice, as needed

1. In a blender, combine the almond milk, pumpkin purée, cashews, Swerve, pumpkin pie spice, and salt and blend until smooth.

2. Add a couple of ice cubes and blend again, adding ice cubes until your desired consistency is reached.

Variation: **Add one cup of fresh spinach to reap all of the amazing health benefits this superfood has to offer.**

Per Serving: **Calories: 263; Total Fat: 19g; Protein: 7g; Total Carbohydrates: 16g; Fiber: 5g; Net Carbs: 11g; Sweetener Carbs: 3g**

Macros: **Fat: 65%; Protein: 11%; Carbs: 24%**

Berry Yogurt Parfaits

SERVES

4

PREP
TIME

15

COOK
TIME

5

This is a grown-up version of a childhood favorite. I like to serve these in individual clear glasses to showcase all the beautiful colors. Raspberries and blackberries are so wonderful for your body, and they are one of the lower-carb fruits. Plain Greek yogurt is thick and full of healthy proteins to help curb your appetite.

½ cup chopped pecans

3 cups plain Greek yogurt

½ teaspoon Swerve granulated sweetener (optional)

1 cup fresh raspberries

1 cup fresh blackberries

1. In a skillet over medium-high heat, toast the pecans for about 5 minutes, until they become one shade darker. Coarsely chop them with a sharp knife and set aside.

2. In a small bowl, mix together the yogurt and Swerve, if using. Spoon ⅓ cup of yogurt into the bottom of each of 4 glasses.

3. Add some of the berries and chopped pecans. Alternate between the yogurt, berries, and pecans until the glasses are full.

Variation: **Transform this into a breakfast smoothie by replacing the pecans with ½ cup of almond milk and blending until well incorporated.**

Per Serving: **Calories: 246; Total Fat: 6g; Protein: 29g; Total Carbohydrates: 19g; Fiber: 5g; Net Carbs: 14g**

Macros: **Fat: 22%; Protein: 31%; Carbs: 47%**

Waffle Batter

30-MINUTE / GLUTEN-FREE / VEGETARIAN

There's no need to bypass waffles on a low-carb diet when you have this recipe up your sleeve. These light and fluffy waffles are perfect for brunch or as a base for a waffle sandwich. The batter is simple to make and you will be amazed that you're eating low-carb. I like to top this with a dollop of nut butter and fresh berries.

SERVES

4

(8 small waffles or
4 large waffles)

PREP
TIME

5

COOK
TIME

5

8 ounces cream cheese, softened

8 large eggs

2 cups almond flour

½ cup Swerve granulated sweetener

4 teaspoons baking powder

½ teaspoon salt

1. Preheat a waffle iron according to the manufacturer's instructions.

2. Add cream cheese, eggs, almond flour, sweetener, baking powder, and salt to a blender and blend until smooth.

3. Pour the batter into the waffle iron and cook until golden brown, according to the manufacturer's instructions.

Variation: If you don't have a waffle maker, you can use this batter to make pancakes.

Per Serving: **Calories: 553; Total Fat: 46g; Protein: 23g; Total Carbohydrates: 13g; Fiber: 4g; Net Carbs: 9g; Sweetener Carbs: 24g**

Macros: **Fat: 75%; Protein: 17%; Carbs: 8%**

Cottage Cheese with Nuts and Berries

30-MINUTE / GLUTEN-FREE / VEGETARIAN

SERVES

4

PREP TIME

5

COOK TIME

2

If you have not tried whipped cottage cheese, you are missing out. This creamy, protein-packed cheese is topped with sweet berries, toasted walnuts, and coconut flakes and will have you craving more. It's healthy, flavorful, and ready in minutes.

4 ounces walnuts, toasted

¼ cup unsweetened coconut flakes, toasted

2 cups full-fat cottage cheese

1 cup sliced strawberries

1 cup blackberries

1. In a small skillet over medium-low heat, toast the walnuts and coconut flakes, stirring consistently for about 2 minutes, until golden brown.

2. In a food processor or blender, pulse the cottage cheese for 2 to 3 minutes, until it is smooth and creamy.

3. Spoon the cottage cheese into individual bowls and top with the berries and toasted nuts.

Variation: **The possibilities are endless with this protein bowl. Change the fruits and nuts to suit your tastes.**

Per Serving: **Calories: 388; Total Fat: 28g; Protein: 19g; Total Carbohydrates: 15g; Fiber: 6g; Net Carbs: 9g**

Macros: **Fat: 65%; Protein: 19%; Carbs: 16%**

Cobb Salad with Poached Eggs

DAIRY-FREE / GLUTEN-FREE

SERVES

4

PREP TIME

15

COOK TIME

20

When was the last time you started your morning with a big ole salad? Packed with fibrous greens, proteins, and healthy fats, this bowl is the perfect way to get your engine revved. If you are a fan of the runny yolk, it serves as the perfect salad dressing. If not, drizzle everything with a little olive oil and freshly squeezed lemon juice.

8 slices bacon, cut into small pieces

10 ounces mixed greens

2 avocados, diced

2 cups halved grape tomatoes

8 large eggs

Salt

Freshly ground black pepper

1. Line a plate with paper towels. In a medium skillet over medium heat, cook the bacon until crispy. Transfer the bacon to the paper towel–lined plate to drain any excess grease.

2. Divide the greens, avocados, and tomatoes among 4 plates and scatter the bacon over the top.

3. In a large saucepan over medium heat, bring 3 inches of water to a gentle simmer.

4. Crack one egg at a time into a small cup, gently add it to the simmering water, and cook for 3 to 5 minutes, until it's done to your liking. Cook 4 eggs at a time. Using a slotted spoon, gently transfer the eggs from the water and place 2 eggs on each salad.

5. Season with salt and pepper and serve.

Variation: **Instead of bacon, use smoked salmon or your favorite cooked fish.**

Per Serving: **Calories: 502; Total Fat: 38g; Protein: 28g; Total Carbohydrates: 14g; Fiber: 7g; Net Carbs: 7g;**

Macros: **Fat: 68%; Protein: 22%; Carbs: 10%**

Brussels Sprout Hash and Cracked Eggs

30-MINUTE / GLUTEN-FREE / ONE-PAN / VEGETARIAN

I took my favorite side dish—Brussels sprouts—and turned it into a healthy, filling breakfast. The combination of sprouts, onions, and bell peppers creates a fresh base that is topped with eggs and Cheddar cheese, resulting in a delicious, low-carb comfort dish.

3 tablespoons
extra-virgin olive oil

4 cups shaved
Brussels sprouts

½ cup chopped onion

½ cup chopped red
bell pepper

1 tablespoon chopped
fresh garlic

8 large eggs

½ cup shredded
Cheddar cheese

¼ teaspoon salt

½ teaspoon freshly
ground black pepper

1. In a large skillet over medium-high heat, warm the olive oil. Add the Brussels sprouts, onion, bell pepper, and garlic and cook for about 10 minutes, until tender.

2. Carefully crack the eggs over the top of the vegetables. Sprinkle with the Cheddar cheese, salt, and pepper.

3. Reduce the heat to low and cover the skillet. Cook for 5 to 6 minutes, until the egg whites are cooked and the cheese is melted.

Simplify it: **To save time, most supermarkets are stocked with pre-shaved Brussels sprouts. If not available, use a food processor to shave the sprouts quickly.**

Per Serving: **Calories: 336; Total Fat: 24g; Protein: 18g; Total Carbohydrates: 12g; Fiber: 4g; Net Carbs: 8g**

Macros: **Fat: 64%; Protein: 21%; Carbs: 15%**

Mediterranean Egg Scramble

30-MINUTE / GLUTEN-FREE / ONE-PAN / VEGETARIAN

Enjoy these soft, creamy eggs with a Mediterranean twist. The pan-fried eggplant in this hearty breakfast stands in for breakfast potatoes and it's tasty enough that you'll never miss them.

SERVES

4

PREP TIME

15

COOK TIME

15

8 large eggs

¼ cup ricotta cheese

2 tablespoons extra-virgin olive oil, plus more for drizzling

1½ cups diced eggplant, peeled (if preferred)

2 teaspoons chopped garlic

¼ cup diced green olives

Salt

Freshly ground black pepper

½ cup diced tomatoes

1. In a mixing bowl, whisk together the eggs and ricotta cheese until well combined. Set aside.

2. In a large skillet over medium-low heat, warm the olive oil for about 30 seconds. Add the eggplant and garlic and cook for 5 to 7 minutes, stirring frequently, until the eggplant is lightly browned and tender.

3. Reduce the heat to low, add the egg mixture and green olives, and cook for about 3 minutes, stirring frequently. Season with salt and pepper.

4. Spoon the mixture into bowls and top each serving with diced tomatoes and a drizzle of olive oil.

Substitution tip: **Replace the ricotta cheese with a bolder cheese like Gorgonzola or provolone for a richer flavor.**

Per Serving: **Calories: 231; Total Fat: 18g; Protein: 13g; Total Carbohydrates: 5g; Fiber: 2g; Net Carbs: 3g**

Macros: **Fat: 70%; Protein: 23%; Carbs: 7%**

Tomato and Spinach Egg Bake

SERVES

4

PREP
TIME

10

COOK
TIME

15

30-MINUTE / GLUTEN-FREE / ONE-PAN / VEGETARIAN

This dish will have you thinking you are eating breakfast at a high-end restaurant. The spinach, cheese, and half-and-half blended together produce a rich, velvety texture that you'll want again and again.

Extra-virgin olive oil or nonstick cooking spray, for greasing the pan

10 ounces fresh baby spinach

4 Roma tomatoes, diced

⅓ cup half-and-half

Salt

Freshly ground black pepper

8 large eggs

½ cup grated Parmesan cheese

1. Preheat the oven to 375°F. Grease a 9-by-12-inch baking dish with olive oil or nonstick cooking spray.

2. Add the spinach to the baking dish and layer the tomatoes on top. Drizzle the half-and-half over the top and season with salt and pepper.

3. Gently crack the eggs over the vegetable mixture and sprinkle with the Parmesan cheese.

4. Bake for 12 to 15 minutes, until the egg whites are opaque.

Variation: **Add cooked breakfast sausage, cooked salmon, or your preferred protein.**

Per Serving: **Calories: 247; Total Fat: 15g; Protein: 19g; Total Carbohydrates: 9g; Fiber: 3g; Net Carbs: 6g**

Macros: **Fat: 55%; Protein: 31%; Carbs: 14%**

Sausage-Stuffed Jalapeños

30-MINUTE / GLUTEN-FREE

The sausage, cream cheese, and Cheddar in this recipe pack a nice punch of protein to give you some morning energy. These are great eaten cold, so make some extras to pack for your lunch the next day.

SERVES

4

PREP TIME

15

COOK TIME

15

8 ounces bulk breakfast sausage

4 ounces cream cheese, softened

¼ cup chopped green onion

½ cup shredded Cheddar cheese

Salt

Freshly ground black pepper

6 medium jalapeños, cut in half lengthwise, seeds removed

1. Preheat the oven to 425°F. Line a baking sheet with foil or parchment paper.

2. In a medium skillet over medium heat, cook the breakfast sausage for about 10 minutes, breaking it up with a spoon while it cooks, until it's browned and cooked throughout. Drain the fat, keeping the sausage in the pan.

3. Reduce the heat to low, add the cream cheese, and stir until well combined. Remove the pan from the heat.

4. Add the green onions and Cheddar cheese to the sausage mixture and stir until combined. Season with salt and pepper.

5. Fill each jalapeño half with the sausage mixture.

6. Place the stuffed jalapeños on the prepared baking sheet and bake for about 20 minutes, until the jalapeños are tender and the cheese is browned.

Variation: **To put a Mediterranean spin on this recipe, use sweet Italian sausage, replace the Cheddar with mozzarella, and replace the green onions with 1 tablespoon of Italian seasoning mix.**

Per Serving: **Calories: 304; Total Fat: 26g; Protein: 15g; Total Carbohydrates: 3g; Fiber: 1g; Net Carbs: 2g**

Macros: **Fat: 77%; Protein: 20%; Carbs: 3%**

Chorizo Frittata

30-MINUTE / GLUTEN-FREE / ONE-POT

Eggs, cheese, and chorizo will start your morning off with a bang. This protein-packed breakfast is bursting with bold flavors and, best of all, it is so simple to make. If you're feeling even more adventurous, chop up a jalapeño instead of the red bell pepper, which will kick up the spice a notch or two.

8 large eggs

⅓ cup half-and-half

¾ cup shredded sharp Cheddar cheese

¼ teaspoon salt

½ teaspoon freshly ground black pepper

8 ounces chorizo

¼ cup diced red bell pepper

1. Preheat the oven to 375°F.

2. In a mixing bowl, whisk together the eggs, half-and-half, Cheddar cheese, salt, and pepper. Set aside.

3. In a cast iron skillet over medium heat, cook the chorizo for 5 to 7 minutes, breaking it up with a spoon, until the chorizo is browned and cooked throughout. Drain any excess grease.

4. Pour the egg mixture over the chorizo and top it with the red bell pepper. Bake for 20 minutes, or until the eggs are set.

Cooking tip: If you don't have a cast iron skillet, use a regular skillet to cook the ingredients and transfer them to a baking dish to bake in the oven.

Per Serving: **Calories: 498; Total Fat: 40g; Protein: 31g; Total Carbohydrates: 3g; Fiber: 0g; Net Carbs: 3g**

Macros: **Fat: 73%; Protein: 25%; Carbs: 2%**

Sheet-Pan Sausage and Veggies

30-MINUTE / DAIRY-FREE / GLUTEN-FREE / ONE-PAN

Roasting ingredients brings out their natural sweetness, leaving you with an elevated burst of flavor and richness. The savory sausage and mushrooms pair well with the sweetness from the asparagus and cherry tomatoes. Together, they make this dish so tasty that it will become a favorite in your low-carb breakfast lineup.

SERVES

PREP
TIME

COOK
TIME

15

Extra-virgin olive oil, for greasing the pan, plus more for drizzling

1 pound breakfast sausage links

2 cups chopped kale

1 cup sliced mushrooms

12 asparagus spears, ends discarded, each cut in half

1 cup cherry tomatoes, halved

Salt

Freshly ground black pepper

1. Preheat the oven to 400° F. Grease a baking sheet with olive oil.

2. Arrange the sausage links, kale, and mushrooms on the baking sheet and drizzle with olive oil. Bake for about 10 minutes, or until the sausage begins to brown.

3. Add the asparagus and tomatoes and bake for an additional 5 to 10 minutes, until the vegetables are tender.

4. Season with salt and pepper.

Variation: **Protein it up by adding eggs to the pan along with the asparagus. You are not limited to just these vegetables, so get creative and use whatever is in season.**

Per Serving: **Calories: 344; Total Fat: 24g; Protein: 22g; Total Carbohydrates: 10g; Fiber: 3g; Net Carbs: 7g**

Macros: **Fat: 63%; Protein: 26%; Carbs: 11%**

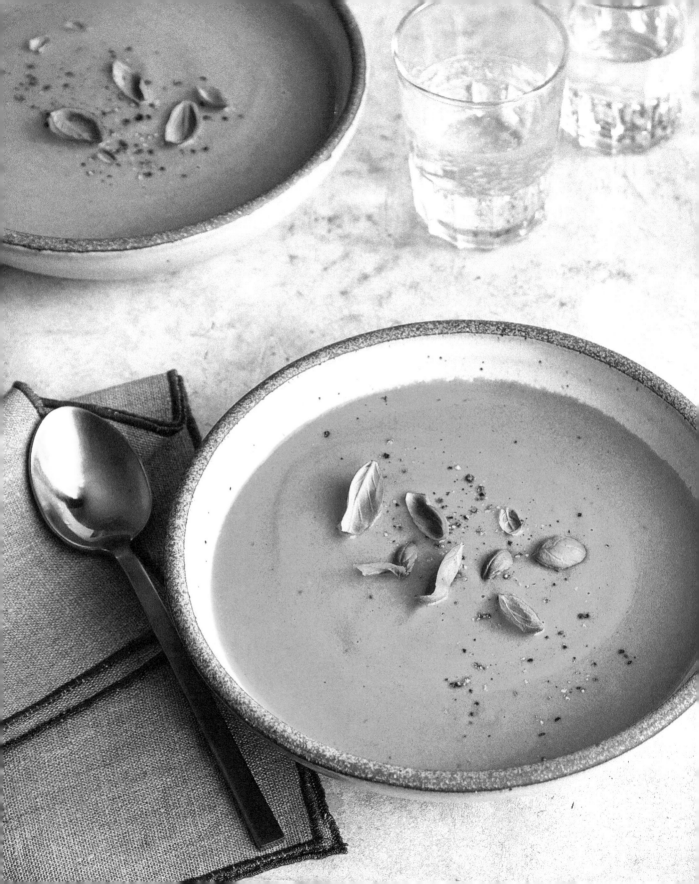

3.

Soups and Salads

Red Pepper Soup

GLUTEN-FREE / VEGETARIAN

SERVES

4

PREP
TIME

15

COOK
TIME

40

This creamy, low-carb soup is packed with flavor and makes an elegant and beautiful first course for a dinner party.

4 red bell peppers

5 garlic cloves, peeled

2 tablespoons extra-virgin olive oil, plus more for drizzling

½ cup chopped onion

4 cups vegetable or chicken stock

3 tablespoons tomato paste

½ cup heavy whipping cream

Salt

Freshly ground black pepper

1. Preheat the oven to 400°F. Line a baking sheet with parchment paper.

2. Place the bell peppers and garlic on the prepared baking sheet and drizzle with olive oil.

3. Bake for 30 minutes, turning the peppers and garlic every 10 minutes to prevent burning, until they are fully roasted.

4. Remove the garlic from the baking sheet and set aside. Transfer the peppers to a bowl, cover, and let sit for 10 minutes. Remove the skin, seeds, and stems and set aside.

5. In a medium stock pot over medium heat, warm 2 tablespoons of olive oil. Add the onions and cook for about 7 minutes, stirring frequently, until they begin to brown.

6. Purée the stock, tomato paste, onions, garlic, and roasted peppers in a blender until smooth. Pour the mixture into the stock pot, add the heavy whipping cream, and season with salt and pepper. Simmer for an additional 10 minutes, until hot.

Simplify it: **Ditch the blender and use a handheld immersion blender to save time.**

Per Serving: **Calories: 243; Total Fat: 19g; Protein: 3g; Total Carbohydrates: 15g; Fiber: 3g; Net Carbs: 12g**

Macros: **Fat: 70%; Protein: 5%; Carbs: 25%**

Roasted Vegetable Soup

GLUTEN-FREE / ONE-POT / VEGAN

This soup will please everyone. The caramelization from browning the vegetables creates a sweet, nutty flavor that will set this hearty soup apart.

SERVES

4

PREP TIME

10

COOK TIME

30

2 tablespoons extra-virgin olive oil

8 ounces fresh green beans, cut into bite-size pieces

10 ounces cauliflower, cut into bite-size pieces

2 tablespoons chopped garlic

8 cups vegetable broth

1 (14.5-ounce) can diced tomatoes

2 cups chopped kale

Salt

Freshly ground black pepper

Chopped fresh herbs, for garnish (optional)

Juice of ½ lemon (optional)

1. In a large stock pot over medium-low heat, warm the olive oil. Add the green beans and cauliflower and cook for 7 to 9 minutes, stirring frequently, until they begin to brown. Add the garlic and cook for an additional 2 minutes, stirring occasionally.

2. Increase the heat to high, add the vegetable broth, diced tomatoes, and kale, and bring to a boil. Reduce the heat to low, cover, and simmer for 15 to 20 minutes, until the vegetables are tender.

3. Season with salt and pepper. Serve with fresh herbs or some freshly squeezed lemon juice (if using) for a pop of flavor.

Variation: **Transform this soup into vegetable-beef soup by searing 2 pounds of chuck steak, cut into ½-inch cubes, before browning the vegetables. Substitute beef or chicken broth for the vegetable broth.**

Per Serving: **Calories: 222; Total Fat: 10g; Protein: 14g; Total Carbohydrates: 19g; Fiber: 6g; Net Carbs: 13g**

Macros: **Fat: 41%; Protein: 25%; Carbs: 34%**

Chicken-Mushroom Soup

30-MINUTE / GLUTEN-FREE / ONE-POT

SERVES

4

PREP
TIME

15

COOK
TIME

15

This nutritious, flavorful, and hearty low-carb soup is one of my go-tos for a busy weeknight dinner. The mushrooms and cream produce a rich, silky broth that's especially comforting during the cooler months.

2 tablespoons
extra-virgin olive oil

1½ pounds chicken
tenderloins, cut into
½-inch pieces

1 large onion, diced

2 cups sliced mushrooms

1 tablespoon
chopped garlic

4 cups chicken broth

2 cups half-and-half

Salt

Freshly ground
black pepper

1. In a stock pot over medium-high heat, warm the olive oil. Add the chicken, onion, mushrooms, and garlic and cook, stirring frequently, until the chicken begins to brown.

2. Add the chicken broth and half-and-half and bring to a simmer. Reduce the heat to medium-low and simmer for about 10 minutes, until the chicken is cooked through. Season with salt and pepper to taste.

Variation: **If you prefer a thicker soup, stir in ½ teaspoon of xanthan gum. Enhance the flavor profile of this soup by adding chopped fresh herbs and low-carb vegetables.**

Per Serving: **Calories: 473; Total Fat: 27g; Protein: 46g; Total Carbohydrates: 12g; Fiber: 3g; Net Carbs: 9g**

Macros: **Fat: 51%; Protein: 39%; Carbs: 10%**

Mediterranean Seafood Stew

30-MINUTE / DAIRY-FREE / GLUTEN-FREE / ONE-POT

This is a super easy seafood stew that you can have on the table in 30 minutes. I call for cod and shrimp in the recipe, but the seafood options you could use are limitless. Try it with mussels, grouper, clams, or anything else you like.

SERVES

4

PREP TIME

15

COOK TIME

15

2 tablespoons extra-virgin olive oil

½ cup chopped onion

1 tablespoon chopped fresh garlic

4 cups seafood or vegetable stock

1 (14-ounce) can diced tomatoes

1 (1-pound) cod fillet, cut into ½-inch pieces

1 pound shrimp, peeled and deveined

Salt

Freshly ground black pepper

1. In a large pot over medium heat, warm the olive oil. Add the onions and garlic and cook for about 5 minutes, until the onions are tender.

2. Add the stock and tomatoes and bring to a simmer. Add the cod and shrimp and simmer for 10 to 15 minutes, until the fish is cooked through. Season with salt and pepper.

Make it vegan: **Use vegetable stock and replace the cod and shrimp with equal amounts of tofu and mushrooms.**

Per Serving: **Calories: 279; Total Fat: 11g; Protein: 37g; Total Carbohydrates: 8g; Fiber: 2g; Net Carbs: 6g**

Macros: **Fat: 35%; Protein: 53%; Carbs: 12%**

Healthy Hearty Chili

DAIRY-FREE / GLUTEN-FREE / ONE-POT

SERVES

PREP
TIME

COOK
TIME

Even after leaving out the beans that bring up the carb count of traditional chilis, this hearty dish will still keep you satisfied for hours. The unsweetened chocolate gives a richer, more complex flavor to this bowl of comfort.

1 pound ground beef
or turkey

1 tablespoon
chopped garlic

1 (28-ounce) can diced
tomatoes

2 tablespoons
chili powder

1½ tablespoons
ground cumin

2 to 3 ounces
unsweetened chocolate

Salt

Freshly ground
black pepper

1. In a large pot over a medium-high heat, cook the ground beef for about 10 minutes, until browned. Drain any excess grease.

2. Add the garlic and cook for an additional 2 minutes. Reduce the heat to low, add the tomatoes, chili powder, cumin, and chocolate and simmer, covered, for about 10 minutes.

3. Season with salt and pepper and serve.

Make it vegan: **Use 2 cups of shelled edamame instead of the beef or turkey. Edamame is readily available in the frozen vegetable department at most supermarkets.**

Per Serving: **Calories: 366; Total Fat: 22g; Protein: 25g; Total Carbohydrates: 17g; Fiber: 8g; Net Carbs: 9g**

Macros: **Fat: 54%; Protein: 27%; Carbs: 19%**

Harvest Salad

GLUTEN-FREE / VEGAN

Roasted acorn squash brings a subtle sweetness to this autumn-themed salad, and the toasted walnuts bring the crunch. The creamy pumpkin vinaigrette enhances the flavors of these simple ingredients.

SERVES

4

PREP
TIME

15

COOK
TIME

50

FOR THE SALAD:

1 acorn squash, halved, seeds removed

Salt

Freshly ground black pepper

Extra-virgin olive oil, for drizzling

½ cup walnut pieces

10 ounces mixed greens

FOR THE VINAIGRETTE:

3 tablespoons pure pumpkin purée

3 tablespoons balsamic vinegar

¾ cup extra-virgin olive oil

Freshly ground black pepper

1. Preheat the oven to 400°F. Line a baking sheet with parchment paper.

2. Cut the acorn squash into ⅓-inch slices and place on the baking sheet. Season with salt and pepper and drizzle with olive oil. Bake for 35 minutes. Flip the squash with a spatula, then bake for an additional 10 to 15 minutes, until tender. Set aside to cool.

3. In a sauté pan over medium heat, toast the walnuts for about 5 minutes, stirring frequently.

4. In a food processor or blender, blend the pumpkin purée, balsamic vinegar, olive oil, and freshly ground black pepper to make a vinaigrette.

5. Divide the mixed greens between 4 plates, top with the roasted squash, sprinkle with the toasted walnuts, and drizzle with the pumpkin vinaigrette.

Variation: **To make this salad a complete meal, add a heart-healthy protein like a lean cut of chicken, a tuna steak, or a salmon fillet.**

Per Serving: Calories: 516; Total Fat: 48g; Protein: 4g; Total Carbohydrates: 17g; Fiber: 4g; Net Carbs: 13g

Macros: Fat: 84%; Protein: 3%; Carbs: 13%

Green Power Salad

SERVES

PREP
TIME

This salad is a powerhouse of wonderfully nutritious ingredients. The avocado brings a creaminess that works well with the crunchiness from the celery and pumpkin seeds, while the zesty lemon dressing hits your mouth with an explosion at the end.

FOR THE DRESSING:

½ cup extra-virgin olive oil

¼ cup freshly squeezed lemon juice

1 teaspoon minced fresh garlic

Salt

Freshly ground black pepper

FOR THE SALAD:

10 ounces mixed greens

2 avocados, diced

1 cup chopped cucumber

1 cup diced celery

½ cup pumpkin seeds

1. To make the dressing: In a small mixing bowl, whisk together the olive oil, lemon juice, and garlic and season with salt and pepper.

2. To make the salad: In a large mixing bowl, toss together the mixed greens, avocados, cucumber, celery, and pumpkin seeds. Drizzle with the dressing and toss well to combine.

Substitution tip: **If you cannot find pumpkin seeds, sunflower seeds are a wonderful alternative.**

Per Serving: **Calories: 489; Total Fat: 45g; Protein: 7g; Total Carbohydrates: 14g; Fiber: 8g; Net Carbs: 6g**

Macros: **Fat: 83%; Protein: 6%; Carbs: 11%**

Simple Greek Salad

30-MINUTE / GLUTEN-FREE / ONE-POT / VEGETARIAN

This pared-down Greek salad puts summer on a plate with a super-fresh showcase of vibrant flavors. The brightness of the lemon, saltiness of the feta cheese, and crunch of the cucumber all come together perfectly.

SERVES

PREP
TIME

2 cucumbers, peeled
and sliced

2 large tomatoes, diced

½ red onion, thinly sliced

¼ cup chopped fresh dill

1 cup crumbled
feta cheese

¼ cup extra-virgin
olive oil

Juice of 1 lemon

Salt

Freshly ground
black pepper

1. In a large mixing bowl, mix together the cucumbers, tomatoes, onion, and dill.

2. Add the feta cheese, olive oil, and lemon juice. Season with salt and pepper, and stir to combine. Refrigerate the salad for at least 1 hour before serving.

Variation: **Make it a full meal by adding some cubed cooked chicken or salmon.**

Per Serving: **Calories: 277; Total Fat: 21g; Protein: 8g; Total Carbohydrates: 14g; Fiber: 3g; Net Carbs: 11g**

Macros: **Fat: 68%; Protein: 12%; Carbs: 20%**

Roasted Veggie Salad

GLUTEN-FREE / VEGAN

SERVES

4

PREP
TIME

15

COOK
TIME
35

The freshly roasted vegetables in this salad remind me of the rustic dishes typically served in the Italian countryside. I like to make this salad with minimum fuss, mixing it together with an uncomplicated combination of lemon juice, olive oil, salt, and pepper to create the most flavorful light dressing.

10 ounces cauliflower, roughly chopped

2½ cups halved mushrooms

8 cloves garlic, peeled

6 tablespoons extra-virgin olive oil, divided

Salt

Freshly ground black pepper

10 ounces mixed greens

2 avocados, cubed

½ cup roasted almonds

Juice of 2 lemons

1. Preheat the oven to 400°F. Line a baking sheet with parchment paper.

2. In a large mixing bowl, combine the cauliflower, mushrooms, and garlic. Drizzle with 2 tablespoons of olive oil and season with salt and pepper. Transfer the vegetables onto the prepared baking sheet.

3. Bake for 25 to 35 minutes, or until slightly browned, tossing the vegetables halfway through.

4. Divide the mixed greens between 4 shallow bowls and add the roasted vegetables, avocados, and almonds. Drizzle with the remaining 4 tablespoons of olive oil and squeeze the juice of ½ lemon onto each salad.

Variation: **Protein this salad up by adding your favorite cooked fish or chicken breasts.**

Per Serving: **Calories: 455; Total Fat: 39g; Protein: 8g; Total Carbohydrates: 18g; Fiber: 10g; Net Carbs: 8g**

Macros: **Fat: 77%; Protein: 7%; Carbs: 16%**

Salmon Superfood Salad

30-MINUTE / GLUTEN-FREE

Not only are salmon, avocado, and walnuts some of the best superfoods for brain health, but they are also full of heart-healthy fats that will fuel your body for hours. The refreshing natural lemon vinaigrette plays well with the salmon and feta, while the avocado brings a creamy texture to round things out.

SERVES

PREP TIME

COOK TIME

FOR THE SALMON:

Extra-virgin olive oil, for greasing the pan

4 (5-ounce) salmon fillets, at room temperature

Salt

Freshly ground black pepper

FOR THE VINAIGRETTE:

½ cup extra-virgin olive oil

2½ tablespoons freshly squeezed lemon juice

¼ teaspoon salt

⅛ teaspoon freshly ground black pepper

FOR THE SALAD:

8 cups mixed greens

2 avocados, diced

½ cup crumbled feta cheese

½ cup roughly chopped walnuts

1. To make the salmon: Preheat the oven to 425°F. Grease a baking sheet with olive oil.

2. Season the salmon with salt and pepper. Place the salmon skin-side down on the baking sheet and bake for 12 to 15 minutes, until cooked through.

3. To make the vinaigrette: In a small bowl, whisk together the olive oil, lemon juice, salt, and pepper.

4. To make the salad: In a large bowl, toss together the greens, avocado, feta cheese, and walnuts. Add the vinaigrette and toss to coat.

5. Divide the salad mixture between 4 bowls and top with the salmon.

Make it vegetarian: **Replace the salmon with edamame.**

Per Serving: **Calories: 767; Total Fat: 64g; Protein: 36g; Total Carbohydrates: 12g; Fiber: 8g; Net Carbs: 4g**

Macros: **Fat: 75%; Protein: 19%; Carbs: 6%**

Bacon and Spinach Salad

DAIRY-FREE / GLUTEN-FREE

SERVES

4

PREP
TIME

20

COOK
TIME

20

The salad dressing is the star of the show here; it's tart, sweet, and has a subtle hint of bacon. The salad is packed with such wonderful flavors and textures that you could eat it as a light meal all by itself.

FOR THE SALAD:

4 large eggs

1 pound bacon, cut into small pieces

10 ounces fresh baby spinach

½ cup thinly sliced red onion

FOR THE DRESSING:

3 tablespoons extra-virgin olive oil

2 tablespoons balsamic vinegar

½ tablespoon minced garlic

Salt

Freshly ground black pepper

1. Place the eggs in a medium pot and cover with 1 inch of cold water. Cover, bring to a boil over high heat, and boil for 7 to 8 minutes. Remove from the heat and let cool for a few minutes. Peel the eggs, cut them into slices, and set them aside.

2. Line a plate with paper towels. In a skillet over medium heat, cook the bacon for 8 to 10 minutes, stirring frequently, until crispy. Transfer the bacon to the paper towel–lined plate. Reserve the bacon grease in the skillet.

3. In a small bowl, whisk together the olive oil, balsamic vinegar, garlic, and 3 tablespoons of the reserved bacon grease. Season with salt and pepper.

4. Divide the spinach between 4 bowls, add the chopped bacon, red onion, and sliced eggs, and drizzle with the salad dressing.

Variation: **Use shrimp or scallops instead of eggs and sauté them in the bacon grease to make this a heartier meal.**

Per Serving: **Calories: 589; Total Fat: 47g; Protein: 36g; Total Carbohydrates: 6g; Fiber: 2g; Net Carbs: 4g**

Macros: **Fat: 72%; Protein: 24%; Carbs: 4%**

Grilled Beef Salad

30-MINUTE / GLUTEN-FREE

This flavorful salad is a meal-in-one. The beef tenderloin, goat cheese, and balsamic dressing produce a flavor profile that's at once savory, salty, and sweet. Topped off with the crunch from the toasted pecans, you have a meal to please any crowd.

SERVES

4

PREP TIME

COOK TIME

FOR THE STEAKS:

4 (5-ounce) beef tenderloin steaks, at room temperature

Salt

Freshly ground black pepper

Extra-virgin olive oil, for drizzling

FOR THE DRESSING:

½ cup extra-virgin olive oil

¼ cup balsamic vinegar

Salt

Freshly ground black pepper

FOR THE SALAD:

10 ounces mixed greens

½ cup chopped toasted pecans

4 ounces goat cheese, crumbled

1. To make the steaks: Preheat a gas or charcoal grill.

2. Season the steaks with salt and pepper and drizzle with olive oil. Grill the steaks to your desired doneness and let them rest for 5 to 7 minutes.

3. To make the dressing: In a small mixing bowl, whisk together the olive oil and balsamic vinegar and season with salt and pepper. Set aside.

4. To make the salad: Divide the mixed greens between 4 plates and top with the pecans and goat cheese.

5. Cut the steaks into slices and divide between the 4 salads. Drizzle the dressing over the top and serve.

Simplify it: **If you don't feel like firing up the grill, these steaks can easily be cooked in a cast iron skillet over medium-high heat. Warm 1 tablespoon of olive oil before adding the steaks to the pan.**

Per Serving: **Calories: 637; Total Fat: 53g; Protein: 36g; Total Carbohydrates: 4g; Fiber: 2g; Net Carbs: 2g**

Macros: **Fat: 75%; Protein: 23%; Carbs: 2%**

Antipasto Salad

SERVES

4

PREP TIME

25

I like to serve this beautiful salad in a large serving bowl and toss it with the Italian herb vinaigrette just prior to serving. With a selection of ingredients typical in an antipasto, the broad range of flavors here will keep your taste buds fully satisfied.

10 ounces romaine lettuce, chopped

1½ pounds salami, thinly sliced

½ pound provolone cheese, chopped

1 (14-ounce) can artichoke hearts, drained and chopped

½ cup extra-virgin olive oil

3 tablespoons freshly squeezed lemon juice

2 tablespoons dried Italian seasoning

1 tablespoon chopped fresh garlic

Salt

Freshly ground black pepper

1. In a large serving bowl, arrange the romaine, salami, provolone cheese, and artichoke hearts.

2. In a small mixing bowl, whisk together the olive oil, lemon juice, Italian seasoning, and garlic. Season with salt and pepper.

3. Just before serving, drizzle the salad dressing over the salad and toss well.

Substitution tip: Jazz up the salad dressing by replacing the lemon juice with red wine vinegar and 1 tablespoon of Dijon mustard, which will create a more robust and creamy dressing.

Per Serving: **Calories: 1074; Total Fat: 86g; Protein: 55g; Total Carbohydrates: 20g; Fiber: 6g; Net Carbs: 14g**

Macros: **Fat: 72%; Protein: 20%; Carbs: 8%**

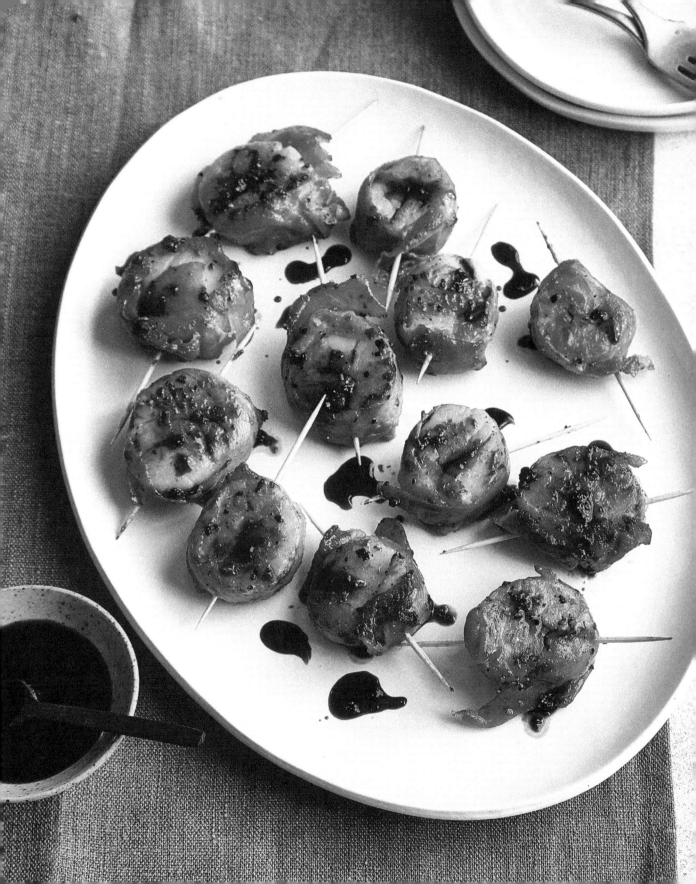

4.

Starters and Sides

Lemony Hummus

30-MINUTE / GLUTEN-FREE / ONE-PAN / VEGAN

SERVES

4

PREP
TIME

10

This is one of my favorite recipes, and I keep it as a staple snack in my refrigerator. The protein-packed chickpeas blended together with the lemon produce a creamy dip with a vibrant citrus flavor.

2 cups canned chickpeas, liquid reserved

½ cup tahini paste

¼ cup extra-virgin olive oil

5 garlic cloves, peeled

Juice of 2 lemons

1 tablespoon ground cumin

Salt

Freshly ground black pepper

1. In a food processor or blender, process the chickpeas, tahini paste, olive oil, garlic, lemon juice, and cumin until smooth. If the hummus is too thick, add some of the reserved chickpea liquid and process until it reaches your desired consistency. Season with salt and pepper.

2. Transfer to a bowl and serve with your favorite raw vegetables.

Variation: **Add 1 tablespoon of chopped fresh jalapeño to spice it up or ¼ cup of drained canned artichoke hearts to change the flavor profile.**

Per Serving: **Calories: 455; Total Fat: 31g; Protein: 13g; Total Carbohydrates: 31g; Fiber: 10g; Net Carbs: 21g**

Macros: **Fat: 61%; Protein: 12%; Carbs: 27%**

Zucchini Fritters

GLUTEN-FREE / VEGETARIAN

Need an excuse to use up an abundance of zucchini? These zucchini fritters make a perfect side dish, appetizer, or even main event in a vegetarian meal. The vibrant flavors of the garlic aioli are a wonderful accompaniment.

SERVES

PREP TIME

COOK TIME

4 cups shredded fresh zucchini

2 teaspoons salt, plus more for seasoning

½ cup almond flour

2 large eggs

½ cup grated Parmesan cheese

10 tablespoons, plus 2 teaspoons mayonnaise, divided

4 garlic cloves, finely minced, divided

2 tablespoons extra-virgin olive oil

1 tablespoon freshly squeezed lemon juice

Freshly ground black pepper

1. Place the shredded zucchini into a colander set over a large bowl. Add the salt, mix well, and let rest for about 10 minutes, until the excess liquid drains. Gently squeeze the zucchini to remove any additional liquid.

2. In a mixing bowl, mix together the zucchini, almond flour, eggs, Parmesan cheese, 2 tablespoons of the mayonnaise, and half of the garlic.

3. Line a large plate with paper towels. In a skillet over medium-high heat, warm the olive oil. Drop the mixture into the skillet, one spoonful at a time, and press each spoonful down with the backside of a spatula to form a patty. Cook for about 3 minutes per side, until the fritters begin to brown. Transfer the fritters to the paper towel–lined plate.

4. In a small mixing bowl, combine the remaining mayonnaise and garlic with the lemon juice to make an aioli. Mix well and season with salt and pepper.

5. Serve the fritters with the aioli on the side for dipping.

Per Serving: **Calories: 499; Total Fat: 47g; Protein: 11g; Total Carbohydrates: 8g; Fiber: 2g; Net Carbs: 6g**

Macros: **Fat: 85%; Protein: 9%; Carbs: 6%**

Green Beans with Blue Cheese

30-MINUTE / GLUTEN-FREE / ONE-PAN / VEGETARIAN

SERVES

4

PREP
TIME

5

COOK
TIME

5

This recipe may turn into one of your go-to side dishes, with the flavors and textures of the green beans, almonds, and cheese all mingling together wonderfully. The dish pairs well with grilled chicken, steak, and fish.

1 tablespoon
extra-virgin olive oil

8 ounces fresh green
beans, trimmed

¼ cup toasted
sliced almonds

Juice of 1 lemon

¼ cup crumbled
blue cheese

Salt

Freshly ground
black pepper

1. In a large skillet over medium-high heat, warm the olive oil. Add the green beans and cook for about 5 minutes, stirring frequently, until tender.

2. Add the almonds and lemon juice and stir to combine.

3. Divide the beans among 4 plates and top each serving with crumbled blue cheese and season with salt and pepper.

Substitution tip: **Broccoli and walnuts also work well in this recipe.**

Per Serving: **Calories: 121; Total Fat: 9g; Protein: 4g; Total Carbohydrates: 6g; Fiber: 3g; Net Carbs: 3g**

Macros: **Fat: 67%; Protein: 13%; Carbs: 20%**

Stuffed Tomatoes Provençal

GLUTEN-FREE / ONE-PAN / VEGETARIAN

Traditional Provençal-style tomatoes are stuffed with garlic, fresh herbs, cheese, and bread crumbs. I have made this low-carb friendly by using riced cauliflower instead of bread crumbs and adding fresh spinach for an extra pop of nutrition. Serve this dish as a side or as a wonderful vegetarian main dish.

SERVES

4

PREP TIME

COOK TIME

Extra-virgin olive oil, for greasing the pan

8 Roma tomatoes

2 cups chopped baby spinach

2 cups riced cauliflower

¾ cup shredded Gruyère cheese, divided

3 garlic cloves, minced

1 tablespoon chopped fresh oregano

Salt

Freshly ground black pepper

1. Preheat the oven to 400°F. Grease a 9-by-13-inch baking pan with olive oil.

2. Cut the tops off of the tomatoes and scoop out the pulp and seeds. Chop the pulp and seeds and set aside.

3. In a mixing bowl, mix together the spinach, cauliflower, ½ cup of Gruyère cheese, garlic, oregano, and about ½ cup of the chopped tomato pulp and seeds. Season with salt and pepper.

4. Spoon the cauliflower mixture into the tomato shells and arrange them in the prepared baking pan.

5. Bake for 20 minutes, or until tender. Sprinkle the tomatoes with the remaining Gruyère cheese and bake for an additional 5 to 7 minutes, or until the cheese is melted.

Simplify it: **Riced cauliflower is conveniently sold in the freezer section of most supermarkets if you don't wish to use a food processor.**

Per Serving: **Calories: 190; Total Fat: 10g; Protein: 10g; Total Carbohydrates: 15g; Fiber: 5g; Net Carbs: 10g**

Macros: **Fat: 47%; Protein: 21%; Carbs: 32%**

Cheesy Lemon Asparagus

30-MINUTE / GLUTEN-FREE / ONE-PAN / VEGETARIAN

SERVES

4

PREP
TIME

5

COOK
TIME

10

This garlic-infused asparagus with browned Parmesan cheese is the ultimate in deliciousness. This side dish is a wonderful accompaniment to just about any steak, fish, or chicken dish.

2 tablespoons extra-virgin olive oil

1 bunch fresh asparagus, trimmed

4 garlic cloves, chopped

1 teaspoon red pepper flakes

Salt

Freshly ground black pepper

½ cup grated Parmesan cheese

Juice of ½ lemon

1. Preheat the oven broiler.

2. In a large oven-safe skillet over medium-high heat, warm the olive oil. Add the asparagus, garlic, and red pepper flakes and cook for about 10 minutes, until the asparagus is crisp yet tender. Season with salt and black pepper.

3. Sprinkle the Parmesan cheese over the asparagus and place under the broiler. Cook until the cheese is browned and bubbly. Drizzle with the lemon juice.

Make it vegan: Omit the cheese and add a second vegetable or some toasted pecans.

Per Serving: **Calories: 130; Total Fat: 10g; Protein: 6g; Total Carbohydrates: 4g; Fiber: 1g; Net Carbs: 3g**

Macros: **Fat: 69%; Protein: 18%; Carbs: 13%**

Herb-Roasted Eggplant

GLUTEN-FREE / ONE-PAN / VEGAN

Roasted eggplant is simple to prepare and so versatile. The key to this dish is to ensure that the fresh herbs and olive oil are liberally coated over every inch of the fleshy side of the eggplant. Eat it alone or topped with your favorite spaghetti sauce and some cheese.

SERVES

PREP TIME

COOK TIME

2 eggplants

Salt

4 tablespoons extra-virgin olive oil

4 teaspoons chopped garlic

2 teaspoons chopped fresh rosemary

2 teaspoons chopped fresh thyme

Freshly ground black pepper

1. Preheat the oven to 400°F. Line a baking sheet with parchment paper.

2. Cut the eggplants in half lengthwise. Cut deep slits in a diamond pattern on the cut side of each eggplant half. Sprinkle with salt and let the eggplant sit for 30 minutes, until it releases any excess liquid. Squeeze the eggplant to remove as much liquid as possible.

3. Drizzle the cut side of the eggplants with the olive oil and season with the garlic, rosemary, thyme, salt, and pepper, making sure that the seasonings get into the deep crevices.

4. Place each half of the eggplant, cut-side down, on the prepared baking sheet and bake for 50 to 60 minutes, or until they are tender.

Per Serving: **Calories: 219; Total Fat: 15g; Protein: 3g; Total Carbohydrates: 18g; Fiber: 10g; Net Carbs: 8g**

Macros: **Fat: 62%; Protein: 5%; Carbs: 33%**

Mushrooms with Horseradish Sauce and Thyme

30-MINUTE / GLUTEN-FREE / ONE-PAN / VEGETARIAN

Garlic, butter, and mushrooms are such an amazing trio, with the mushrooms soaking up the flavors of any ingredient they are cooked with. This dish pairs perfectly with a juicy steak, roasted chicken, or served atop fried cauliflower rice. I prefer to use baby portabella mushrooms, for their meatiness.

½ cup sour cream

¼ cup prepared horseradish

Salt

Freshly ground black pepper

1 tablespoon extra-virgin olive oil

2 tablespoons butter

1 pound mushrooms, stems removed

1 tablespoon chopped fresh garlic

1 tablespoon chopped fresh thyme

Juice of ½ lemon

1. In a small bowl, mix together the sour cream and horseradish and season with salt and pepper.

2. In a large sauté pan over medium-high heat, warm the olive oil and butter. Add the mushrooms and cook for 5 minutes, stirring often. Stir in the garlic and thyme and cook for an additional 2 minutes. Stir in the lemon juice and season with salt and pepper.

3. Serve the mushrooms with the creamy horseradish sauce on the side.

Make it vegan: **Omit the butter and replace the sour cream with your favorite vegenaise and an extra squeeze of lemon juice.**

Per Serving: **Calories: 196; Total Fat: 16g; Protein: 5g; Total Carbohydrates: 8g; Fiber: 2g; Net Carbs: 6g**

Macros: **Fat: 73%; Protein: 10%; Carbs: 17%**

Roasted Acorn Squash with Balsamic and Thyme

GLUTEN-FREE / ONE-PAN / VEGAN

The flavors of this side dish remind me of a little piece of pie. Acorn squash has a mildly sweet flavor that's amplified when roasted with the sweet-tangy flavor of balsamic vinegar. Together, they create a pleasing, but not overwhelming, sweet flavor profile. This dish is great on its own, as a topping for a salad, or as a side dish with fish or poultry.

1 acorn squash, halved, seeded, and cut into ½-inch wedges

¼ cup extra-virgin olive oil

3 tablespoons balsamic vinegar

2 teaspoons fresh thyme

Salt

Freshly ground black pepper

1. Preheat the oven to 400°F. Line a baking sheet with parchment paper.

2. In a large bowl, toss the squash with the olive oil, balsamic vinegar, and thyme, and season with salt and pepper. Transfer the squash to the prepared baking sheet.

3. Bake for 30 to 40 minutes, or until browned and fork tender.

Variation: **Make this a hearty sheet-pan meal by adding some chicken thighs and Brussels sprouts. Season them with salt and pepper, drizzle them with olive oil, and bake them along with the squash until the chicken is cooked through.**

Per Serving: **Calories: 177; Total Fat: 13g; Protein: 1g; Total Carbohydrates: 14g; Fiber: 2g; Net Carbs: 12g**

Macros: **Fat: 66%; Protein: 2%; Carbs: 32%**

Spaghetti Squash

GLUTEN-FREE / ONE-PAN / VEGETARIAN

SERVES

4

PREP
TIME

5

COOK
TIME

60

Serve this as a side dish instead of pasta. The squash has a subtle sweetness that pairs well with fresh herbs and olive oil. Top it with spaghetti sauce or serve it in place of rice or mashed potatoes. I promise you—it is a true crowd-pleaser.

1 (2- to 2½-pound) spaghetti squash, cut in half lengthwise

Salt

Freshly ground black pepper

2 tablespoons extra-virgin olive oil, plus more for drizzling

1 tablespoon chopped fresh basil

1 tablespoon chopped fresh parsley

1 teaspoon chopped fresh rosemary

2 garlic cloves, chopped

¼ cup grated Parmesan cheese

1. Preheat the oven to 400°F. Line a baking sheet with parchment paper.

2. Season the cut side of the squash with salt and pepper and drizzle it with olive oil.

3. Place the squash, cut-side down, on the prepared baking sheet and bake for 50 to 60 minutes, or until tender. Let cool for a few minutes.

4. Using a fork, scrape the spaghetti squash strands into a mixing bowl. Add the olive oil, basil, parsley, rosemary, and garlic and mix well to combine. Season with salt and pepper.

5. Transfer the mixture to a serving bowl and sprinkle with Parmesan cheese.

Simplify it: **The squash can be cooked in a slow cooker set on high for 3 to 5 hours or on low for 6 to 8 hours.**

Per Serving: **Calories: 174; Total Fat: 10g; Protein: 4g; Total Carbohydrates: 17g; Fiber: 1g; Net Carbs: 16g**

Macros: **Fat: 52%; Protein: 9%; Carbs: 39%**

Zesty Fish Ceviche

DAIRY-FREE / GLUTEN-FREE / ONE-POT

Ceviche is a fresh, low-carb dish where the seafood is "cooked" in citrus juices, and it only takes minutes to prepare. Light and zesty, the dish can be served in a bowl or in a classic martini glass when entertaining. Choose any fresh whitefish you'd like—my favorites are bass, cod, halibut, tilapia, or snapper.

SERVES

PREP TIME

COOK TIME

1 pound fresh whitefish, cut into ¼-inch pieces and chilled

1½ cups diced tomatoes, seeds removed

1 cup fresh lime juice

¾ cup chopped cilantro

¼ cup minced red onion

Salt

Freshly ground black pepper

1. In a glass or stainless-steel bowl, mix together the fish, tomatoes, lime juice, cilantro, and onion and season with salt and pepper.

2. Cover and let the mixture marinate in the refrigerator for at least 4 hours, or until the fish becomes firmer and opaque in appearance.

Variation: Add ¼ cup of fresh orange juice and two tablespoons of minced jalapeño to add a hint of sweet and spicy.

Per Serving: **Calories: 108; Total Fat: 1g; Protein: 21g; Total Carbohydrates: 4g; Fiber: 1g; Net Carbs: 3g**

Macros: **Fat: 8%; Protein: 77%; Carbs: 5%**

Salmon and Avocado Bites

30-MINUTE / DAIRY-FREE / GLUTEN-FREE

SERVES

4

PREP TIME

30

The red onion mashed together with the avocado adds a subtle bite that works well against the smokiness of the salmon in this dish. Serve these bites at your next brunch or as a quick lunch that can be ready in minutes. Easy, light, and healthy!

1 large avocado, mashed

2 tablespoons minced red onion

1 tablespoon chopped fresh dill

Salt

Freshly ground black pepper

1 or 2 cucumbers, cut into ¼-inch slices

8 ounces smoked salmon, cut into bite-size pieces

Freshly squeezed lemon juice, for garnish

Extra-virgin olive oil, for drizzling

1. In a small bowl, mix together the avocado, red onion, and dill until incorporated. Season with salt and pepper.

2. Assemble the individual bites by spreading the avocado blend onto a slice of cucumber and topping it with some smoked salmon. Repeat with the remaining cucumber slices.

3. Garnish with pepper, lemon juice, and a drizzle of olive oil.

Variation: **Swap the avocado out for cream cheese and wrap the salmon around small pieces of pickled asparagus for a different flavor profile.**

Per Serving: **Calories: 178; Total Fat: 9g; Protein: 12g; Total Carbohydrates: 10g; Fiber: 4g; Net Carbs: 6g**

Macros: **Fat: 51%; Protein: 27%; Carbs: 22%**

Salmon Croquettes

30-MINUTE / GLUTEN-FREE

The simplicity of the ingredients in this recipe allows the salmon to really shine. These croquettes can be served as an appetizer, or you can make it a meal by adding them to the top of a garden-fresh salad.

SERVES

4

PREP TIME

15

COOK TIME

15

1 (1-pound) salmon fillet

½ cup water

Juice of 1 lemon, divided

Salt

Freshly ground black pepper

2 large eggs

⅓ cup mayonnaise

½ cup grated Parmesan cheese

½ cup almond flour

½ tablespoon minced fresh garlic

2 tablespoons extra-virgin olive oil, for frying

1. In a sauté pan over medium heat, place the salmon skin-side down. Add the water and half of the lemon juice, and season with salt and pepper. Cover the pan, bring to a simmer, and cook for about 10 minutes, until the salmon is cooked through. Transfer the salmon to a plate and let it cool.

2. Remove the skin and shred the salmon.

3. In a mixing bowl, mix together the salmon, eggs, mayonnaise, Parmesan cheese, almond flour, garlic, and the remaining lemon juice until combined. Using your hands, form the mixture into 8 (2½-inch) patties.

4. In a skillet over medium heat, warm the olive oil. Add the patties and cook for about 2 minutes on each side, until golden brown.

Substitution tip: **Canned salmon or canned tuna can also be used for this recipe.**

Per Serving: **Calories: 398; Total Fat: 28g; Protein: 33g; Total Carbohydrates: 3g; Fiber: 1g; Net Carbs: 2g**

Macros: **Fat: 63%; Protein: 33%; Carbs: 4%**

Prosciutto-Wrapped Sea Scallops with Balsamic Glaze

15

30-MINUTE / DAIRY-FREE / GLUTEN-FREE

The balsamic glaze immediately hits with a hint of sweetness, followed by the prosciutto's crispy saltiness, and rounded out by the scallop's creamy texture and subtle hint of the sea. Pair these scallops with a steak for a surf-and-turf night. You will need wooden toothpicks to secure the prosciutto around the scallops.

½ cup balsamic vinegar

2 teaspoons Swerve brown sugar substitute

1 teaspoon grated fresh ginger

12 large sea scallops

Salt

Freshly ground black pepper

12 slices prosciutto

1 tablespoon extra-virgin olive oil

1. In a saucepan over medium-high heat, bring the balsamic vinegar, Swerve, and ginger to a slow simmer and cook for about 5 minutes, until the sauce reduces and becomes syrupy. Set aside.

2. Season the scallops with salt and pepper. Wrap each scallop with a slice of prosciutto and secure it with a toothpick, if needed.

3. In a sauté pan over medium-high heat, warm the olive oil. Add the scallops to the pan and cook for about 2 minutes per side, until slightly browned.

4. Remove the toothpicks and divide the scallops between 4 plates. Serve with the balsamic syrup glaze on the side or drizzle the glaze on top of each scallop before serving.

Substitution tip: **Bacon can be used in place of the prosciutto, and shrimp works well in place of the scallops.**

Per Serving: **Calories: 344; Total Fat: 16g; Protein: 42g; Total Carbohydrates: 8g; Fiber: 0g; Net Carbs: 8g; Sweetener Carbs: 2g**

Macros: **Fat: 42%; Protein: 49%; Carbs: 7%**

Pork-Stuffed Mushrooms

DAIRY-FREE

Think of these as a low-carb version of potstickers from your favorite Chinese restaurant. By replacing the wonton wrapper with a mushroom, this popular finger food transforms into a healthy alternative.

SERVES

4

PREP TIME

15

COOK TIME

25

20 to 24 medium mushrooms

2 tablespoons extra-virgin olive oil

1 teaspoon minced fresh garlic

2 teaspoons grated fresh ginger

1 pound ground pork

1 tablespoon soy sauce

2 teaspoons sesame oil

Salt

Freshly ground black pepper

1. Preheat the oven to 375°F. Line a baking sheet with parchment paper.

2. Remove and chop the stems of the mushrooms and set them aside. Using a spoon, scoop out the gills and discard.

3. In a skillet over medium heat, warm the olive oil. Add the garlic and mushroom stems and cook, stirring, until the mushrooms are tender. Add the ginger and cook for an additional minute. Remove from the heat and let cool.

4. In a large mixing bowl, mix together the ground pork, soy sauce, sesame oil, and mushroom stems and season the mixture with salt and pepper.

5. Arrange the mushroom caps on the prepared baking pan. Fill each cap with a spoonful of the pork and mushroom mixture.

6. Bake for 20 to 25 minutes, or until the internal temperature of the pork is 160°F.

Variation: Transform these into Italian stuffed mushrooms by omitting the soy sauce, sesame oil, and ginger and replacing them with Italian seasoning, Parmesan cheese, and 1 large egg.

Per Serving: **Calories: 350; Total Fat: 26g; Protein: 24g; Total Carbohydrates: 5g; Fiber: 1g; Net Carbs: 4g**

Macros: **Fat: 67%; Protein: 27%; Carbs: 6%**

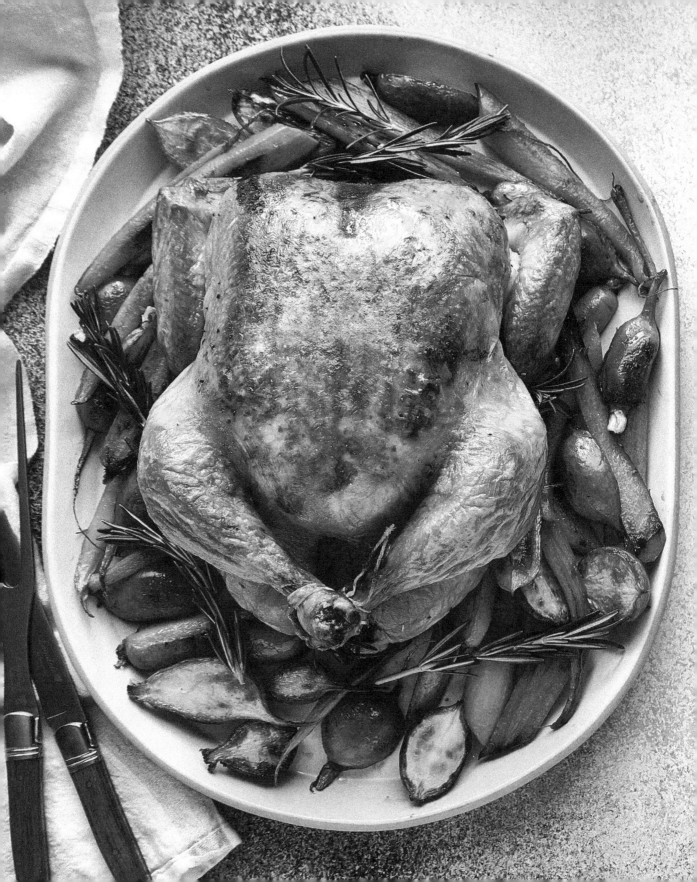

5.

Seafood and Poultry Mains

< Orange-Rosemary Roasted Chicken, *page 76*

Scallop and Asparagus with Zoodles

30-MINUTE / GLUTEN-FREE / ONE-PAN

This classic seafood dish is light, fresh, and delicate in flavor. The garlic, wine, and butter come together to create a savory pan sauce that works perfectly with the tender scallops and asparagus. Serve this over a bed of zoodles with freshly grated Parmesan cheese.

4 tablespoons extra-virgin olive oil, divided

1 pound asparagus, cut into ½-inch pieces

3 tablespoons butter

4 garlic cloves, minced

½ cup dry white wine or seafood broth

2 pounds large sea scallops

Juice of ½ lemon

6 cups spiralized zucchini or zucchini ribbons

1. In a large sauté pan over medium-high heat, warm 2 tablespoons of olive oil. Add the asparagus and sauté for 4 to 5 minutes, until cooked. Transfer to a separate bowl and set aside.

2. In the same pan, add the butter, remaining olive oil, and garlic and sauté for about 1 minute, until the garlic is fragrant. Add the wine, bring to a simmer, stirring well, and cook for 2 more minutes. Add the scallops and cook for 2 to 3 minutes on each side.

3. Return the asparagus to the pan and stir in the lemon juice. Add the zucchini and it let sit for 1 to 2 minutes, covered, until warmed through.

Variation: **This is a standard scampi recipe that can be used for almost any fish or vegetable. It's also nice with shellfish like mussels, clams, or lobster tails.**

Per Serving: **Calories: 465; Total Fat: 25g; Protein: 43g; Total Carbohydrates: 17g; Fiber: 5g; Net Carbs: 12g**

Macros: **Fat: 48%; Protein: 37%; Carbs: 15%**

Shrimp and Cauliflower Grits

30-MINUTE / GLUTEN-FREE

Shrimp and grits are a staple comfort dish in the South. The creamy cauliflower works perfectly as a low-carb substitute for traditional grits. Cooking the shrimp in a small amount of bacon grease adds an additional "Southern" touch.

SERVES

PREP TIME

COOK TIME

1 pound large shrimp, peeled and deveined

2 teaspoons chopped garlic

Salt

Freshly ground black pepper

4 cups riced cauliflower

1½ cups half-and-half

1 cup shredded Cheddar cheese

4 slices bacon, chopped

Green onion, sliced, for garnish (optional)

Paprika, for garnish (optional)

Cayenne pepper, for garnish (optional)

1. Season the shrimp with garlic, salt, and pepper and set aside.

2. In a saucepan over medium-low heat, mix together the cauliflower and half-and-half and bring to a simmer. Cook for about 10 minutes, until the cauliflower is tender. Add the Cheddar cheese, season with salt and pepper, and cook for 5 minutes, stirring often.

3. Line a plate with paper towels. In a large skillet over medium heat, cook the bacon until it reaches your desired doneness. Transfer the bacon to the paper towel–lined plate. Reserve 1 tablespoon of the bacon grease in the skillet and discard the rest.

4. Increase the heat to medium-high, add the shrimp to the skillet, and cook for about 2 minutes per side, stirring occasionally, until the shrimp is pink.

5. Spoon the cauliflower "grits" into bowls and top with the shrimp. Sprinkle with the bacon. If you'd like, garnish with green onion, paprika, or cayenne pepper (if you are feeling adventurous).

Per Serving: **Calories: 469; Total Fat: 29g; Protein: 42g; Total Carbohydrates: 10g; Fiber: 3g; Net Carbs: 7g**

Macros: **Fat: 56%; Protein: 36%; Carbs: 8%**

Shrimp Caprese

30-MINUTE / GLUTEN-FREE / ONE-PAN

SERVES

4

PREP
TIME

10

COOK
TIME

10

One-skillet meals are the best for a weeknight after a long, busy day. Here, I've taken the traditional caprese salad and transformed it into a full meal. The addition of the shrimp, balsamic vinegar, and melted cheese completely transforms this dish from delicious to outstanding.

1 pound large shrimp, peeled and deveined

½ cup halved grape tomatoes

½ cup cubed fresh mozzarella cheese

¼ cup chopped fresh basil

1 tablespoon balsamic vinegar

1 teaspoon chopped garlic

2 tablespoons extra-virgin olive oil

Salt

Freshly ground black pepper

1. Preheat the oven to 400°F. Line a baking sheet with parchment paper.

2. In a mixing bowl, mix together the shrimp, tomatoes, mozzarella cheese, basil, balsamic vinegar, garlic, and olive oil. Season with salt and pepper.

3. Spread the mixture onto the prepared baking sheet and bake for 8 to 10 minutes, or until the shrimp is pink.

4. Set the oven to broil. Broil until the cheese browns.

Variation: **Go ahead and use scallops instead of shrimp. I also like to add a base of fresh spinach to the baking sheet before adding the shrimp and cooking as instructed. Then you won't have to worry about preparing an additional vegetable side dish.**

Per Serving: **Calories: 211; Total Fat: 11g; Protein: 26g; Total Carbohydrates: 2g; Fiber: 0g; Net Carbs: 2g**

Macros: **Fat: 47%; Protein: 49%; Carbs: 4%**

Mediterranean Cod

30-MINUTE / GLUTEN-FREE / ONE-PAN

Anytime I can get my hands on some cod, I'm all over it. Cod has a dense, white, flaky flesh with a mild taste that pairs well with many flavors. Like most fish, it cooks quickly, and it's nice to eat something so delicious knowing that it's also healthy.

SERVES

PREP TIME

10

COOK TIME

15

½ tablespoon chopped fresh garlic

½ tablespoon dried oregano

¼ teaspoon salt

⅛ teaspoon freshly ground black pepper

4 (5-ounce) cod fillets

2 tablespoons plus 4 teaspoons extra-virgin olive oil

½ cup pitted green olives

½ cup pitted Kalamata olives

8 tablespoons crumbled feta cheese

Juice of 1 lemon

1. In a small bowl, mix together the garlic, oregano, salt, and pepper and rub it over both sides of the cod fillets.

2. In a large skillet over medium heat, warm 2 tablespoons of olive oil. Add the cod and cook for 4 to 5 minutes on each side, until the internal temp reaches 145°F. Turn the heat off.

3. Add the green and Kalamata olives to the pan, cover, and let sit for about 2 minutes.

4. Place 1 cod fillet on each of 4 plates and spoon the olives equally over each plate. Top each with 2 tablespoons of feta cheese, 1 teaspoon of olive oil, and the lemon juice.

Variation: **One pound of peeled and deveined shrimp works well in place of the cod.**

Per Serving: **Calories: 330; Total Fat: 22g; Protein: 28g; Total Carbohydrates: 5g; Fiber: 2g; Net Carbs: 3g**

Macros: **Fat: 60%; Protein: 34%; Carbs: 6%**

Tilapia with Tomatoes and Wine Sauce

30-MINUTE / GLUTEN-FREE / ONE-PAN

The flavor profile of this dish is elevated, but it's quite simple to prepare; just be sure to use a dry white wine like sauvignon blanc, pinot grigio, or pinot gris. Serve this alongside my Stuffed Tomatoes Provençal (see page 49) or Cheesy Lemon Asparagus (see page 50).

4 (5-ounce) tilapia fillets, at room temperature

Salt

Freshly ground black pepper

2 tablespoons extra-virgin olive oil

1 cup halved cherry or grape tomatoes

1 garlic clove, chopped

1 cup dry white wine

4 tablespoons cold butter

¼ cup chopped fresh basil

1 lemon, quartered, for serving

1. Season the tilapia with salt and pepper.

2. In a large nonstick skillet over medium-high heat, warm the olive oil. Add the tilapia fillets and cook for 3 to 5 minutes per side. Transfer the fillets to a plate and cover to keep warm.

3. Add the tomatoes and garlic to the pan and cook for about 3 minutes, stirring often to prevent burning. Add the wine, bring the mixture to a simmer, and cook for an additional 5 minutes. Using a whisk, release any browned bits from the bottom of the pan—this will add more flavor to the sauce.

4. Reduce the heat to low and whisk in the butter until melted and emulsified. Stir in the basil. Serve with ¼ of a lemon on each plate to squeeze over the top.

Ingredient tip: Tilapia is a delicate fish, so it's best to use a nonstick pan. I also like to cut the butter into four pieces and add them one at a time for better emulsification into the sauce.

Per Serving: Calories: 304; Total Fat: 20g; Protein: 27g; Total Carbohydrates: 4g; Fiber: 1g; Net Carbs: 3g

Macros: Fat: 59%; Protein: 36%; Carbs: 5%

Cajun Grouper with Alfredo Sauce

30-MINUTE / GLUTEN-FREE / ONE-PAN

SERVES

4

PREP
TIME

10

COOK
TIME

20

Grouper is a mild whitefish that is very meaty and holds up well to any bold flavor profile. My Cajun Seasoning (page 131) makes this dish special; paired with a creamy alfredo sauce, the hint of spice makes this a very comforting meal.

4 (5-ounce) grouper fillets, at room temperature

8 ounces Cajun Seasoning (see page 131) or store-bought

2 tablespoons extra-virgin olive oil

2 tablespoons butter

2 teaspoons minced garlic

1½ cups heavy whipping cream

½ cup grated Parmesan cheese

Salt

Freshly ground black pepper

Juice of 1 lemon

1. Season the grouper with the Cajun seasoning.

2. In a large skillet over medium-high heat, warm the olive oil. Add the grouper fillets and cook on each side for 3 to 6 minutes, depending on the thickness of the fillets. Transfer to a plate and set aside.

3. Lower the temperature to medium and let the skillet sit for about 5 minutes. Add the butter and the garlic and cook until the garlic begins to soften. Add the heavy whipping cream, bring to a low simmer, and cook for about 5 minutes, stirring, until the sauce begins to reduce and thicken.

4. Stir in the Parmesan cheese and cook for an additional 3 to 5 minutes.

5. Season with salt and pepper, add more Cajun seasoning if you prefer more heat. Plate your fish, top with sauce, and drizzle with lemon juice.

Make it vegetarian: **Replace the grouper with an assortment of sliced vegetables, such as zucchini, mushrooms, bell peppers, or asparagus.**

Per Serving: **Calories: 617; Total Fat: 50g; Protein: 38g; Total Carbohydrates: 4g; Fiber: 0g; Net Carbs: 4g**

Macros: **Fat: 73%; Protein: 25%; Carbs: 2%**

Tuna Poke Bowls

SERVES

PREP
TIME

It doesn't get any fresher than this dish. This traditional Hawaiian bowl is virtually carb-free and bursting with so many island flavors. You will love it.

2 pounds sushi-grade ahi tuna, cut into ½-inch cubes

1 cup thinly sliced green onion

1 cup soy sauce

¼ cup sesame oil

1 tablespoon grated fresh ginger

Salt

Freshly ground black pepper

1. In a bowl, mix together the tuna, green onion, soy sauce, sesame oil, and ginger. Season with salt and pepper.

2. Cover and refrigerate for at least 2 hours before serving.

Substitution tip: **To make this dish gluten-free, use coconut aminos or gluten-free tamari instead of soy sauce.**

Per Serving: **Calories: 375; Total Fat: 16g; Protein: 50g; Total Carbohydrates: 8g; Fiber: 1g; Net Carbs: 7g**

Macros: **Fat: 38%; Protein: 53%; Carbs: 9%**

Seafood Medley

Go ahead and get creative with this recipe and customize it with whatever seafood is freshest at the grocery store. I'm a big fan of cod, snapper, grouper, or bass, but feel free to choose your favorite varieties. Buttered spinach serves as a perfect accompaniment to any seafood medley.

SERVES

4

PREP TIME

10

COOK TIME

10

1 pound large shrimp, peeled and deveined

1 pound firm whitefish, cubed, at room temperature

Salt

Freshly ground black pepper

1 tablespoon extra-virgin olive oil

4 tablespoons butter

¼ cup chopped garlic

16 ounces baby spinach

Freshly squeezed lemon juice, for garnish

1. Season the shrimp and fish with salt and pepper.

2. In a large sauté pan over medium-high heat, warm the olive oil. Add the fish and cook for 5 minutes, stirring. Add the shrimp and continue to cook, approximately 3 to 5 minutes more, stirring, until cooked throughout. Remove from the pan and set aside.

3. Add the butter and garlic and cook, stirring, for about 1 minute. Add the spinach, season with salt and pepper, and stir until the spinach begins to wilt. Turn off the heat.

4. Divide the spinach between 4 plates and top it with the shrimp and fish. Drizzle with the lemon juice.

Simplify it: **To save time on prepping, purchase peeled and deveined shrimp from your seafood freezer section. Most supermarkets also sell frozen seafood medley packages.**

Per Serving: **Calories: 382; Total Fat: 18g; Protein: 48g; Total Carbohydrates: 7g; Fiber: 3g; Net Carbs: 4g**

Macros: **Fat: 42%; Protein: 50%; Carbs: 8%**

Snapper and Vegetables
en Papillote

30-MINUTE / DAIRY-FREE / GLUTEN-FREE / ONE-PAN

En papillote is a method of cooking in which the food is put into a sealed pouch then baked. The ingredients are steamed, trapping all the fresh flavors within the envelope. Serve this light, low-carb dish with a fresh salad for the ideal balanced dinner.

4 (6-ounce) snapper fillets

Salt

Freshly ground black pepper

8 ounces fresh spinach

4 cups julienned fresh zucchini

¾ cup halved cherry or grape tomatoes

8 fresh thyme sprigs

4 teaspoons chopped fresh garlic

4 teaspoons extra-virgin olive oil

1 or 2 fresh lemons, sliced

1. Preheat the oven to 375°F. Have a baking sheet and 4 sheets of aluminum foil or parchment paper ready.

2. Season the snapper fillets with salt and pepper.

3. Divide the ingredients between the 4 sheets of foil in this order: spinach, snapper, zucchini, tomatoes, thyme, garlic, olive oil, and lemon slices.

4. Seal the individual packets and place them on the baking sheet. Bake for 12 to 15 minutes, depending on the thickness of the fish.

5. Serve in the packet, being careful of any hot steam when opening.

Variation: **Experiment with different fish, vegetables, and herbs for this dish. One of my favorite combinations is salmon, asparagus, mushrooms, and dill.**

Per Serving: **Calories: 296; Total Fat: 8g; Protein: 47g; Total Carbohydrates: 9g; Fiber: 3g; Net Carbs: 6g**

Macros: **Fat: 24%; Protein: 64%; Carbs: 12%**

Sun-Dried Tomato–Stuffed Chicken

GLUTEN-FREE / ONE-PAN

SERVES

4

PREP TIME

15

COOK TIME

30

The sun-dried tomatoes paired with the creaminess of the provolone create a wonderfully complementary sweet and smoky flavor in this dish. Have some wooden toothpicks on hand to seal the chicken.

4 boneless, skinless chicken breasts

Salt

Freshly ground black pepper

4 slices provolone cheese, each cut in half

10 ounces fresh baby spinach, divided

8 tablespoons chopped sun-dried tomatoes in olive oil

1 tablespoon extra-virgin olive oil

1½ cups heavy whipping cream

2 teaspoons minced garlic

1. Preheat the oven to 375°F.

2. Butterfly the chicken breasts by cutting each one almost all the way through horizontally and opening it like a book. Season with salt and pepper.

3. On one side of each butterflied chicken breast, layer ½ slice of provolone cheese, a handful of spinach, 2 tablespoons of sun-dried tomatoes, and another ½ slice of cheese. Seal with toothpicks.

4. In a large cast iron skillet over medium-high heat, warm the olive oil. Add the stuffed chicken breasts and sear for about 4 minutes per side, until golden.

5. Add the heavy whipping cream and garlic and season with salt and pepper. Bake for 20 to 25 minutes, or until the internal temperature of the chicken reaches 165°F.

6. Transfer the chicken to a platter and set aside. Add the remaining spinach and cook, stirring, until the spinach wilts.

7. Divide the spinach sauce between 4 plates and top each with a stuffed chicken breast.

Per Serving: Calories: 637; Total Fat: 49g; Protein: 38g; Total Carbohydrates: 11g; Fiber: 3g; Net Carbs: 8g

Macros: Fat: 69%; Protein: 24%; Carbs: 7%

Chili-Lime Chicken

DAIRY-FREE / GLUTEN-FREE / ONE-PAN

SERVES

MARINATE
TIME

PREP
TIME

10

COOK
TIME

35

If you want chicken that is jam-packed with flavor, then this recipe is calling your name. The chili powder gives it a little kick, and the fresh lime juice brightens everything up with a pop of freshness.

½ cup chopped cilantro

3 tablespoons chili powder

2 tablespoons Swerve brown sugar sweetener

Juice of 4 limes

3 tablespoons chopped garlic

¼ cup extra-virgin olive oil

Salt

Freshly ground black pepper

2 pounds chicken thighs

1. In a large resealable plastic bag, mix together the cilantro, chili powder, Swerve, lime juice, garlic, olive oil, salt, and pepper.

2. Add the chicken thighs, seal the bag tightly, and refrigerate for at least 2 (and up to 24) hours.

3. Preheat the oven to 375°F.

4. Remove the chicken from the marinade and let it come to room temperature for about 20 minutes.

5. In a large oven-safe skillet over medium-high heat, add the chicken, skin-side down, and sear for about 5 minutes on each side, until browned.

6. Transfer the pan to the oven and bake for 20 to 25 minutes, or until the internal temperature reaches 165°F.

Variation: **This recipe also works well with beef. Make the recipe with sliced skirt steak and use it in fajitas.**

Per Serving: **Calories: 632; Total Fat: 48g; Protein: 41g; Total Carbohydrates: 9g; Fiber: 2g; Net Carbs: 7g; Sweetener Carbs: 6g**

Macros: **Fat: 68%; Protein: 26%; Carbs: 6%**

Smoky Chicken with Roasted Brussels Sprouts

GLUTEN-FREE / ONE-PAN

This is a great one-pan dinner to make on a busy weeknight. The prep time is short and then you pop it into the oven, giving you time to tend to other things while it cooks. It's also impressive enough to serve to guests.

SERVES

4

PREP TIME

15

COOK TIME

45

4 chicken drumsticks

Salt

Freshly ground black pepper

1 pound Brussels sprouts, trimmed

¼ cup extra-virgin olive oil, plus more for drizzling

4 tablespoons butter

1 tablespoon smoked paprika

¼ cup chopped fresh parsley

3 garlic cloves, minced

1. Preheat the oven to 375°F. Line a sheet pan with parchment paper.

2. Season the drumsticks with salt and pepper. Set aside.

3. Place the Brussels sprouts on the prepared sheet pan. Season them with salt and pepper, drizzle with olive oil, and toss well.

4. In a small saucepan over medium-low heat, mix together the butter, olive oil, smoked paprika, parsley, and garlic, and cook for 1 to 2 minutes.

5. In a mixing bowl, add the chicken, pour in the butter mixture, and toss to coat evenly. Transfer the chicken to the sheet pan, placing them throughout the Brussels sprouts. Drizzle any remaining sauce over the chicken and vegetables.

6. Bake for 35 to 45 minutes, or until the internal temperature of the chicken reaches 165°F.

Per Serving: **Calories: 512; Total Fat: 40g; Protein: 26g; Total Carbohydrates: 12g; Fiber: 5g; Net Carbs: 8g**

Macros: **Fat: 70%; Protein: 20%; Carbs: 10%**

Roasted Chicken and Leek Gravy

GLUTEN-FREE / ONE-PAN

This dish is all about the caramelized leek gravy. The leeks absorb all of the flavor of the chicken since they are at the base of the pan. Roasting the leeks produces a sweet and nutty flavor that pairs well with the chicken flavor. Serve this alongside your favorite sautéed vegetables, such as asparagus or green beans.

4 skin-on chicken thighs

Salt

Freshly ground
black pepper

2 tablespoons
extra-virgin olive oil,
plus more for drizzling

1 large leek, thinly sliced

8 whole garlic
cloves, peeled

1 tablespoon fresh thyme

1 cup chicken stock

¼ to ½ cup heavy
whipping cream

1. Preheat the oven to 400°F. Line a baking sheet with parchment paper.

2. Season the chicken with the salt and pepper and drizzle with olive oil.

3. Remove the dark green top and the root from the leek, then cut the leek lengthwise into quarters. Rinse each piece in a water-filled sink. Drain and set aside.

4. Slice the leek and place it on the prepared baking sheet. Scatter the garlic and thyme over the top. Season with salt and pepper, drizzle with olive oil, and toss to combine. Place the chicken on top of the leek mixture.

5. Bake for 40 to 45 minutes, or until the internal temperature of the chicken reaches 165°F. Transfer the chicken to a serving plate and set aside.

6. In a blender, purée the vegetable mixture, pan drippings, and chicken stock until creamy and transfer the mixture to a saucepan. Add the heavy whipping cream slowly until the mixture reaches the consistency of alfredo sauce. Simmer the sauce over medium-low heat for about 5 minutes, until heated through. Season with salt and pepper.

7. Serve the chicken with the gravy poured over the top.

Simplify it: **If you have an immersion blender, purée the gravy in the saucepan instead of transferring the sauce to a blender.**

Per Serving: **Calories: 455; Total Fat: 39g; Protein: 19g; Total Carbohydrates: 7g; Fiber: 1g; Net Carbs: 6g**

Macros: **Fat: 77%; Protein: 17%; Carbs: 6%**

Orange-Rosemary Roasted Chicken

DAIRY-FREE / GLUTEN-FREE / ONE-PAN

Orange and rosemary are a great combination, and they infuse the chicken from the inside out. The orange juice also helps keep the chicken moist.

2 tablespoons chopped fresh rosemary, plus 3 to 4 sprigs

1 orange, zested and quartered

12 garlic cloves, peeled, divided

3 tablespoons extra-virgin olive oil, plus more for drizzling

2 teaspoons salt, divided

2½ teaspoons freshly ground black pepper, divided

1 pound radishes, trimmed

12 ounces carrots, peeled and halved

1 (6- to 7-pound) whole roasting chicken

1. Preheat the oven to 400°F. Have a roasting pan ready.

2. In a food processor or blender, process 2 table-spoons of rosemary, the orange zest, 4 of the garlic cloves, the olive oil, 1 teaspoon of salt, and ½ teaspoon of pepper, until minced.

3. Place the radishes, carrots, and 4 more garlic cloves in the roasting pan. Season with ½ teaspoon of salt and ½ teaspoon of pepper and drizzle with olive oil. Place the chicken on the vegetables, breast side up.

4. Gently loosen the skin of the chicken and evenly rub the herb mixture underneath the skin. Season the outside of the chicken with the remaining salt and pepper. Add the orange quarters, rosemary sprigs, and the remaining garlic cloves inside the chicken cavity.

5. Roast for 1½ to 2 hours, or until the internal temperature reaches 165°F.

Per Serving: **Calories: 543; Total Fat: 32g; Protein: 42g; Total Carbohydrates: 21g; Fiber: 6g; Net Carbs: 15g**

Macros: **Fat: 53%; Protein: 31%; Carbs: 16%**

Chicken and Cauliflower Steaks Provolone

GLUTEN-FREE

SERVES

4

PREP TIME

20

COOK TIME

20

In this low-carb twist on a classic comfort dish, cauliflower steaks bring a meaty texture with plenty of flavor from when they are browned during cooking.

2 tablespoons extra-virgin olive oil, divided, plus more for greasing the pan

1 pound chicken cutlets

1 small head cauliflower, cut into ¼-inch slices

Salt

Freshly ground black pepper

3 garlic cloves, chopped

1 teaspoon Italian seasoning

1½ cups canned crushed tomatoes

4 to 6 slices provolone cheese

1. Preheat the oven to 425°F. Lightly grease an 8-by-8-inch baking dish with olive oil.

2. Season the chicken and cauliflower steaks with salt, pepper, garlic, and Italian seasoning.

3. In a skillet over medium-high heat, warm 1 tablespoon of olive oil. Add the cauliflower steaks and sear on each side for 2 to 3 minutes, or until slightly browned and tender. Transfer to a plate and set aside.

4. In the same skillet over medium-high heat, add the remaining olive oil and the chicken cutlets, and cook for about 3 minutes per side. Set aside with the cauliflower.

5. Place the chicken in the prepared baking dish. Add half of the crushed tomatoes, half of the provolone cheese, the cauliflower steaks, followed by the remaining crushed tomatoes and cheese.

6. Bake for 15 to 20 minutes, or until the cheese is browned.

Per Serving: **Calories: 388; Total Fat: 20g; Protein: 40g; Total Carbohydrates: 13g; Fiber: 5g; Net Carbs: 8g**

Macros: **Fat: 46%; Protein: 41%; Carbs: 13%**

Chicken-Mushroom Melts

30-MINUTE / GLUTEN-FREE

SERVES

4

PREP
TIME

10

COOK
TIME

20

The combination of the mushrooms, chicken, bacon, and Cheddar cheese create a deceptively low-carb bite. Add a tablespoon of your favorite low-carb honey mustard to replicate a favorite recipe from a familiar Aussie steakhouse.

4 chicken breasts, at room temperature

Salt

Freshly ground black pepper

Extra-virgin olive oil, for drizzling

8 slices bacon

1 cup sliced mushrooms

1 cup shredded Cheddar cheese

1. Preheat a gas or charcoal grill.

2. Season the chicken breasts with salt and pepper and drizzle with olive oil.

3. Line a plate with paper towels. In a skillet over medium heat, cook the bacon to your desired crispness and set aside on the prepared plate. Reserve 1 tablespoon of the bacon fat in the skillet.

4. In the same skillet over medium heat, warm the bacon grease. Add the mushrooms and cook for about 8 minutes, until tender. Season with salt and pepper. Set aside.

5. Grill the chicken breasts for 7 to 8 minutes per side, or until the internal temperature reaches 165°F.

6. Preheat the broiler. Have a baking sheet ready.

7. Place the chicken on the baking sheet. Top with mushrooms, strips of bacon, and sprinkle with the Cheddar cheese. Broil until the cheese melts.

Make it vegetarian: **Replace the chicken breast with a cauliflower steak.**

Per Serving: **Calories: 473; Total Fat: 30g; Protein: 48g; Total Carbohydrates: 2g; Fiber: 0g; Net Carbs: 2g**

Macros: **Fat: 57%; Protein: 41%; Carbs: 2%**

Shawarma-Style Turkey

DAIRY-FREE / GLUTEN-FREE

Turkey breast tenderloins are incredibly tender and offer a generous amount of meat. The flavors of this marinade are quite bold and absolutely delicious. When cooked on the grill, the paprika and cumin infuse a wonderful smokiness into the turkey. Serve with my Simple Greek Salad (see page 37), Lemony Hummus (see page 46), or Tzatziki Sauce (see page 130).

SERVES

4

MARINATE TIME

2hr

PREP TIME

10

COOK TIME

40

½ cup extra-virgin olive oil

¼ cup freshly squeezed lemon juice

5 garlic cloves, minced

2 teaspoons ground cumin

2 teaspoons paprika

1 teaspoon salt

1 teaspoon freshly ground black pepper

¾ teaspoon ground turmeric

½ teaspoon ground nutmeg

1½ to 2 pounds turkey breast tenderloins

1. In a large resealable plastic bag, add the olive oil, lemon juice, garlic, cumin, paprika, salt, pepper, turmeric, and nutmeg and mix well. Add the turkey, seal the bag, and refrigerate for at least 2 (and up to 24) hours.

2. Preheat a gas or charcoal grill to medium heat.

3. Remove the turkey and let it come to room temperature, reserving the marinade.

4. Grill for 35 to 40 minutes, turning occasionally and basting with the reserved marinade, until the internal temperature reaches 165°F.

Simplify it: **Cook the recipe in a slow cooker to save time and energy. Place the turkey into the slow cooker with ½ cup of the marinade and cook it on low for 5 to 6 hours, or until it reaches an internal temperature of 165°F.**

Per Serving: **Calories: 475; Total Fat: 27g; Protein: 55g; Total Carbohydrates: 3g; Fiber: 1g; Net Carbs: 2g**

Macros: **Fat: 51%; Protein: 46%; Carbs: 3%**

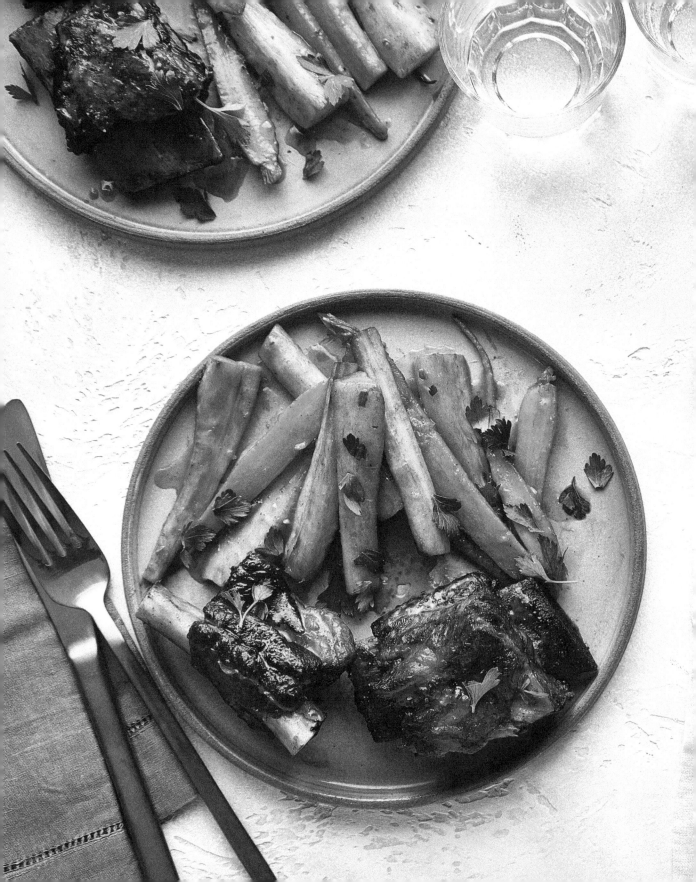

6.

Pork, Lamb, and Beef Mains

< Red Wine Beef Short Ribs with Carrots and Parsnips, *page 98*

Carnitas with Coleslaw

DAIRY-FREE / GLUTEN-FREE

SERVES

4

PREP
TIME

15

COOK
TIME

5hr

This is an ideal meal for Taco Tuesday. The pork shoulder can be placed into the slow cooker early in the morning, and it will be ready by the time everyone gets home at the end of the day.

1½ tablespoons chili powder, divided

2 tablespoons ground cumin

1½ teaspoons salt, divided

2½ teaspoons freshly ground black pepper, divided

1 (3- to 4-pound) pork shoulder

6 teaspoons chopped garlic, divided

Juice of 2 oranges, divided

4 cups shredded cabbage

½ tablespoon extra-virgin olive oil

1. In a small bowl, mix together 1 tablespoon of chili powder, the cumin, 1 teaspoon of salt, and 2 teaspoons of pepper. Rub the seasoning all over the pork shoulder.

2. Place 5 teaspoons of chopped garlic, the juice of 1 orange, and the seasoned pork shoulder into a slow cooker. Cover and cook for 8 hours on low or 4 to 5 hours on high. The meat should fall apart when cooked properly.

3. Transfer the pork shoulder to a cutting board, shred the meat, and return it to the pot along with any juices. Season with salt and pepper and cover.

4. Preheat the oven to broil.

5. Place the shredded pork on a baking sheet and broil for 3 to 4 minutes, until crispy.

6. In a mixing bowl, combine the cabbage with the remaining orange juice, chili powder, and garlic and the olive oil. Mix well and season with the remaining salt and pepper.

Substitution tip: **Not a fan of pork? You can easily swap it out for skinless chicken thighs for an equally satisfying result.**

Per Serving: **Calories: 920; Total Fat: 72g; Protein: 59g; Total Carbohydrates: 9g; Fiber: 4g; Net Carbs: 5g**

Macros: **Fat: 70%; Protein: 26%; Carbs: 4%**

Rosemary Pork Roast

DAIRY-FREE / GLUTEN-FREE

By using the vegetables in this dish as a roasting bed, they absorb the luscious flavors from the pork drippings. The vegetables can be served as is or puréed with the pan drippings as a rich gravy to complement the roast and the other vegetables.

SERVES

4

PREP
TIME

10

COOK
TIME

3hr

¼ cup chopped fresh rosemary

¼ cup chopped garlic

3 tablespoons extra-virgin olive oil, divided

1 teaspoon salt

½ teaspoon freshly ground black pepper

2 cups whole mushrooms, trimmed

2 cups turnips, cut into cubes

1 head cabbage, cut into 8 wedges

1 (2- to 2½-pound) pork shoulder roast

¾ cup water

1. Preheat the oven to 450°F.

2. In a mixing bowl, mix together the rosemary, garlic, 2 tablespoons of olive oil, salt, and pepper into a paste.

3. In a large baking dish, toss together the mushrooms, turnips, and cabbage. Season the vegetables with salt and pepper and drizzle with the remaining olive oil.

4. Score the top of the pork roast in a crosshatch pattern and set it on top of the vegetable mixture. Generously rub the rosemary mixture over the entire surface of the roast. Add the water to the baking dish.

5. Roast for 20 minutes. Cover with aluminum foil, reduce the oven temperature to 325°F, and cook for 3 hours, or until the internal temperature reaches 160°F.

Simplify it: **Instead of manually chopping the ingredients for the paste, purée them in a blender until smooth.**

Per Serving: **Calories: 765; Total Fat: 57g; Protein: 43g; Total Carbohydrates: 20g; Fiber: 8g; Net Carbs: 12g**

Macros: **Fat: 67%; Protein: 22%; Carbs: 11%**

Caribbean Pork Ribs and Cauliflower Rice

DAIRY-FREE / GLUTEN-FREE

SERVES

4

PREP
TIME

15

COOK
TIME

2½hr

Caribbean cuisine is known for its bold and rich flavors, and this recipe follows suit. Seasoned with curry powder, cumin, and the sweetness of Swerve brown sugar, you'll want to make these anytime you are in the mood for a tropical vacation.

2 racks baby back ribs

¼ cup Swerve brown sugar sweetener

3 tablespoons curry powder, divided

3 tablespoons minced garlic, divided

3 tablespoons extra-virgin olive oil, divided

1½ tablespoons ground cumin, divided

Salt

Freshly ground black pepper

1 head cauliflower, riced

Juice of ½ lemon

1. Preheat the oven to 300°F. Line a baking sheet with aluminum foil.

2. Remove the membrane from the backside of the ribs. In a small bowl, mix together the Swerve, 2 tablespoons of curry powder, 2 tablespoons of garlic, 2 tablespoons of olive oil, 1 tablespoon of cumin, salt, and pepper. Generously rub the ribs with the mixture.

3. Add the ribs to the prepared baking sheet. Cover with another sheet of aluminum foil and bake for 2 to 2½ hours, or until the meat falls off the bone.

4. In a large skillet over medium-high heat, warm the remaining 1 tablespoon of olive oil. Add the remaining 1 tablespoon of garlic and cook for 30 seconds. Add the riced cauliflower, remaining 1 tablespoon of curry powder, and remaining ½ tablespoon of cumin and cook for 5 minutes. Pour in the lemon juice, stir, and continue to cook for an additional 3 minutes.

5. Serve the ribs alongside the cauliflower rice.

Per Serving: **Calories: 521; Total Fat: 33g; Protein: 45g; Total Carbohydrates: 11g; Fiber: 3g; Net Carbs: 8g; Sweetener Carbs: 12g**

Macros: **Fat: 57%; Protein: 35%; Carbs: 8%**

Pork with Bacon, Apple, and Brussels Sprouts

30-MINUTE / DAIRY-FREE / GLUTEN-FREE

Bacon, pork, apples, and Brussels sprouts make one of my favorite combinations that I frequently serve in my kitchen. Inspired by German cuisine, this hearty and comforting dish will keep you satisfied for hours.

6 cups Brussels sprouts, trimmed and halved

¼ pound bacon, chopped

1 small onion, sliced

½ red apple, peeled and chopped

3 garlic cloves, chopped

2 tablespoons extra-virgin olive oil, divided

2½ teaspoons salt, divided

1½ teaspoons freshly ground black pepper, divided

1 (2- to 2½-pound) pork tenderloin

1. Preheat the oven to 425°F. Line a baking sheet with parchment paper.

2. In a mixing bowl, combine the Brussels sprouts, bacon, onion, apple, garlic, and 1 tablespoon of olive oil. Mix well and season with ½ teaspoon of salt and ½ teaspoon of pepper.

3. Season the pork tenderloin with the remaining salt and pepper and drizzle with the remaining olive oil. Place it in the center of the baking sheet. Spread the Brussels sprouts mixture around the pork.

4. Bake for 30 minutes, or until the internal temperature of the pork reaches 145°F.

Substitution tip: Shredded cabbage can be substituted for the Brussels sprouts, and chicken can be used in place of the pork.

Per Serving: Calories: 544; Total Fat: 24g; Protein: 63g; Total Carbohydrates: 19g; Fiber: 7g; Net Carbs: 12g

Macros: Fat: 40%; Protein: 46%; Carbs: 14%

Pork with Green Beans and Apricot Relish

SERVES

4

MARINATE
TIME

24hr

PREP
TIME

20

COOK
TIME

35

Pork shoulder steaks are nicely marbled with fat, which greatly enhances their flavor. Pork and fruit always pair together to create a powerhouse flavor profile. Since this entire meal is cooked over the grill, you will find that cleanup is a breeze.

¼ cup plus 1 teaspoon balsamic vinegar, divided

1 tablespoon plus ½ teaspoon fresh thyme, divided

5 tablespoons chopped garlic, divided

1 teaspoon salt

½ teaspoon freshly ground black pepper

3 tablespoons plus 1 teaspoon extra-virgin olive oil, plus more for drizzling

1 to 1½ pounds pork shoulder steaks

1 cup halved and pitted fresh apricots

1 pound fresh green beans, trimmed

2 tablespoons water

1. In a large resealable bag, mix together ¼ cup of balsamic vinegar, 1 tablespoon of thyme, 4 tablespoons of garlic, salt, pepper, and 3 tablespoons of olive oil. Add the pork steaks, seal the bag, and refrigerate for up to 24 hours.

2. Preheat a gas or charcoal grill to medium-high heat.

3. Season the apricots with salt and pepper and drizzle with olive oil.

4. Place the green beans on a large sheet of foil and add 1 teaspoon of olive oil, the remaining garlic, and the water. Seal the sides of the foil to form a pouch.

5. Remove the pork shoulder steaks from the marinade and let them sit at room temperature for 20 minutes.

6. Grill the pork for 5 to 7 minutes per side, until the internal temperature reaches 160°F. Transfer to a plate and let rest for 10 minutes.

7. Add the green bean pouch to the grill over direct heat and cook for 10 to 15 minutes, turning the pouch halfway through, until tender. Season with salt and black pepper.

8. Place the apricots, cut-side down, directly on the grill rack and grill for 1 minute. Turn them over and grill for an additional 30 seconds. Remove the skin, dice, and mix with the remaining 1 teaspoon of balsamic vinegar and ½ teaspoon of thyme. Season with salt and pepper.

9. Serve the steaks topped with the apricot relish and with the green beans on the side.

Variation: **Many fruits can be grilled and paired with this recipe. Try peaches, plums, pears, or pineapple. But remember—eat fruit in moderation because they tend to be higher in carbs.**

Per Serving: **Calories: 469; Total Fat: 30g; Protein: 33g; Total Carbohydrates: 18g; Fiber: 5g; Net Carbs: 13g**

Macros: **Fat: 58%; Protein: 28%; Carbs: 14%**

Sesame Pork and Bok Choy

DAIRY-FREE

SERVES

4

MARINATE
TIME

2hr

PREP
TIME

20

COOK
TIME

30

Bok choy is a Chinese cabbage that is low in calories and high in vitamins. The lean pork tenderloin married with the bok choy makes a healthy and flavorful meal.

¼ cup soy sauce, plus more for drizzling

2 tablespoons grated fresh ginger, divided

3 teaspoons minced garlic, divided

3 tablespoons extra-virgin olive oil, divided

1 teaspoon salt, divided

1½ teaspoons freshly ground black pepper, divided

1 (1½- to 2-pound) lean pork tenderloin

¼ cup sesame seeds

1½ pounds baby bok choy, cut in half lengthwise

1. In a large resealable plastic bag, mix together the soy sauce, 1½ tablespoons of ginger, 2 teaspoons of garlic, 1 tablespoon of olive oil, ½ teaspoon of salt, and 1 teaspoon of pepper. Add the pork tenderloin, seal the bag, and refrigerate for at least 2 hours.

2. Preheat the oven to 400°F. Have a 9-by-13-inch baking dish ready. Remove the pork from the marinade and let it sit at room temperature for at least 20 minutes.

3. Place the sesame seeds in a large shallow bowl. Drizzle the pork loin with 1 tablespoon of olive oil and roll it in the sesame seeds, coating evenly.

4. Place the pork tenderloin into the baking dish and bake for 20 minutes, or until the internal temperature reaches 145°F. Let it rest for 10 minutes.

5. In a large skillet over medium-high heat, warm the remaining 1 tablespoon olive oil. Add the remaining 1 teaspoon of garlic and ½ tablespoon of ginger and cook for about 30 seconds, until they become fragrant. Add the bok choy and cook for 5 to 7 minutes, stirring occasionally, until they begin to brown. Season with the remaining salt and black pepper.

6. Drizzle the bok choy with soy sauce and serve alongside the pork.

Per Serving: Calories: 425; Total Fat: 23g; Protein: 46g; Total Carbohydrates: 9g; Fiber: 3g; Net Carbs: 6g

Macros: Fat: 49%; Protein: 43%; Carbs: 8%

Sweet and Sour Pork Chops

DAIRY-FREE / GLUTEN-FREE

This meal will easily become your low-carb replacement for take-out sweet and sour pork. Add this to your next Sunday night dinner lineup, and don't hesitate to make extras for lunch during the week.

SERVES

4

PREP
TIME

10

COOK
TIME

40

4 (5-ounce) pork chops, at room temperature

Salt

Freshly ground black pepper

2 tablespoons extra-virgin olive oil, divided

1 tablespoon chopped garlic

4 cups sliced red, yellow, or orange bell peppers

Juice of 1 orange

2 tablespoons Swerve brown sugar sweetener

2 tablespoons apple cider vinegar

1. Season each side of the pork chops with salt and black pepper.

2. In a large skillet over medium-high heat, warm 1 tablespoon of olive oil. Add the pork chops and cook for 5 minutes. Turn them over, cover the pan, and cook for 2 more minutes, until the temperature reaches 145°F. Transfer to a plate and set aside.

3. Add the remaining olive oil to the skillet. Add the garlic and bell peppers and cook for 5 to 7 minutes, until the peppers begin to brown.

4. Add the orange juice, Swerve, and apple cider vinegar and cook for 3 to 5 minutes, until the sauce begins to reduce. Season with salt and black pepper.

5. Divide the pork chops between 4 plates and top with the bell pepper sauce.

Make it vegan: **Instead of pork, use tofu steaks, which will absorb the flavors of this dish very nicely.**

Per Serving: **Calories: 387; Total Fat: 27g; Protein: 25g; Total Carbohydrates: 12g; Fiber: 3g; Net Carbs: 9g; Sweetener Carbs: 6g**

Macros: **Fat: 63%; Protein: 26%; Carbs: 11%**

Homemade Italian Sausage Patties

4

PREP
TIME

15

COOK
TIME

15

30-MINUTE / GLUTEN-FREE

This homemade version of Italian sausage is free of sugars and other added fillers often found in commercial versions. The fennel seeds add a slight licorice flavor and are a traditional ingredient used in Italian cuisine. Make these patties in bulk and freeze them individually to have on standby for an easy meal.

1 pound ground pork

8½ cups baby spinach, divided, ½ cup chopped

½ cup grated Parmesan cheese, plus more for topping

1 tablespoon Italian seasoning

½ teaspoon fennel seeds

2 garlic cloves, grated and divided

1½ teaspoons salt, divided

2½ teaspoons freshly ground black pepper, divided

1 tablespoon extra-virgin olive oil

1. In a mixing bowl, mix the ground pork, ½ cup of chopped spinach, Parmesan cheese, Italian seasoning, fennel seeds, half of the garlic, 1 teaspoon of salt, and 2 teaspoons of pepper. Form the mixture into 4 patties.

2. In a large skillet over medium-high heat, warm the olive oil. Add the sausage patties and cook for 5 to 7 minutes, until they are nicely browned and have reached an internal temperature of 160°F. Transfer to a plate and set aside.

3. Reduce the heat to medium and add the remaining spinach and garlic to the skillet. Mix well to incorporate and season with the remaining salt and pepper. Place the sausage patties on top of the spinach, cover, and cook for 1 to 2 minutes.

4. Divide the spinach between 4 plates and top with the sausages. Sprinkle additional Parmesan cheese over the top and serve.

Per Serving: **Calories: 407; Total Fat: 32g; Protein: 26g; Total Carbohydrates: 5g; Fiber: 2g; Net Carbs: 3g**

Macros: **Fat: 71%; Protein: 26%; Carbs: 3%**

Lamb Gyro Lettuce Boats

30-MINUTE / GLUTEN-FREE / ONE-PAN

There's no need to hit your local Greek takeaway the next time you're craving a gyro. Traditionally, the meat is cooked on a vertical rotisserie for hours, but here you can get the same flavors in 30 minutes.

SERVES

4

PREP TIME

15

COOK TIME

15

1 pound ground lamb

1 tablespoon chopped garlic, divided

½ tablespoon chopped fresh oregano

Juice of 1 lemon, divided

3 teaspoons extra-virgin olive oil, divided

¾ teaspoon salt

¾ teaspoon freshly ground black pepper

½ cup plain Greek yogurt

8 romaine lettuce leaves, plus 2 cups shredded romaine

½ cup crumbled feta cheese

1. In a mixing bowl, mix together the ground lamb, ½ tablespoon of garlic, oregano, half of the lemon juice, 2 teaspoons of olive oil, salt, and pepper.

2. In a skillet over medium-high heat, warm the remaining olive oil. Add the ground lamb mixture and cook until browned and cooked throughout, about 8 minutes. Remove from the heat.

3. In a mixing bowl, mix together the Greek yogurt and the remaining garlic and lemon juice, and season the mixture with salt and pepper.

4. Place 2 lettuce leaves on each of 4 plates. Assemble the lettuce boats in this order: ground lamb, shredded lettuce, feta cheese, Greek yogurt sauce.

Substitution tip: If ground lamb is not readily available, ground beef can be used instead.

Per Serving: Calories: 463; Total Fat: 35g; Protein: 31g; Total Carbohydrates: 6g; Fiber: 1g; Net Carbs: 5g

Macros: Fat: 68%; Protein: 28%; Carbs: 4%

Lamb Chops with Lemon-and-Mint Asparagus

SERVES

4

MARINATE
TIME

4hr

PREP
TIME

15

COOK
TIME

15

This recipe offers a low-carb take on the classic combination of lamb and mint. Here, the lamb chops work well against the fresh and vibrant flavors from the lemon-and-mint asparagus. Serve this with my Simple Greek Salad (see page 37).

3 tablespoons chopped fresh oregano

Juice of 1½ lemons, divided

¼ cup plus 2 tablespoons extra-virgin olive oil, divided, plus more for drizzling

4 tablespoons grated garlic, divided

2 teaspoons salt, divided

2½ teaspoons freshly ground black pepper, divided

8 (3- to 4-ounce) bone-in lamb loin chops

1 pound asparagus, trimmed

1½ teaspoons chopped fresh mint

1. In a resealable plastic bag, mix together the oregano, juice of 1 lemon, ¼ cup of olive oil, 3 tablespoons of garlic, 1 teaspoon of salt, and 2 teaspoons of pepper. Add the lamb chops, seal the bag, and refrigerate for at least 4 (and up to 12) hours.

2. Remove the lamb from the marinade, pat dry, and let it sit at room for 20 minutes.

3. In a skillet over medium-high heat, add 1 tablespoon of olive oil. Add the lamb chops and cook for 4 to 6 minutes per side. Transfer to a plate and let rest.

4. Wipe out the skillet and over medium-high heat, warm the remaining 1 tablespoon of olive oil. Add the asparagus and sauté for 4 to 5 minutes, until fork tender. Add the remaining 1 tablespoon of garlic and sauté for 1 more minute. Add the mint, remaining lemon juice, 1 teaspoon of salt, and ½ teaspoon of pepper.

5. Divide the lamb chops and asparagus between 4 plates and drizzle with olive oil.

Per Serving: **Calories: 529; Total Fat: 37g; Protein: 38g; Total Carbohydrates: 11g; Fiber: 5g; Net Carbs: 6g**

Macros: **Fat: 63%; Protein: 29%; Carbs: 8%**

Beef and Bacon Lettuce Boats

30-MINUTE / GLUTEN-FREE / ONE-POT

Peppered bacon is the star of this dish. It has become quite popular and is readily available at most grocery stores. However, if you can't find it, you can use regular bacon and coat it with pepper prior to cooking. These flavorful lettuce boats make a great lunch or a quick dinner on busy weeknights.

SERVES

PREP TIME

COOK TIME

8 slices peppered bacon, chopped

1½ pounds ground beef

Salt

8 romaine lettuce leaves

½ cup crumbled blue cheese

½ cup diced fresh tomatoes

1. Line a plate with paper towels. In a large skillet over medium-low heat, cook the bacon until browned and crispy. Transfer to the paper towel–lined plate to drain. Reserve 1 tablespoon of the bacon grease in the skillet.

2. Add the ground beef to the skillet and cook, stirring occasionally, over medium-high heat for 8 to 10 minutes, until browned and cooked throughout. Drain any excess grease and season with salt.

3. Place 2 lettuce leaves on each of 4 plates. Layer the ingredients in this order: ground beef, blue cheese, tomatoes, and chopped bacon.

Variation: **Transform these into Mexican-flavored tacos with lettuce "tortillas" by omitting the bacon, seasoning the beef with 2 tablespoons of chili powder and 1 tablespoon of ground cumin, and topping them with salsa and Cheddar cheese.**

Per Serving: **Calories: 511; Total Fat: 33g; Protein: 51g; Total Carbohydrates: 2g; Fiber: 0g; Net Carbs: 2g**

Macros: **Fat: 58%; Protein: 40%; Carbs: 2%**

Ribeye with Sautéed Mushrooms and Onions

30-MINUTE

Have you ever wondered why a steak always tastes best in a steak house? The key is in the high-heat cooking and simple seasoning, plus a little finishing butter. First, get a quick char on the steak by seasoning it with salt, and then baste the steak with butter as it cooks to your desired doneness. The secret is out!

4 (5-ounce) rib eye steaks, at room temperature

Salt

Freshly ground black pepper

2 tablespoons extra-virgin olive oil, divided

4 tablespoons butter

2 garlic cloves, chopped

4 cups sliced mushrooms

1 medium onion, sliced

1 tablespoon Worcestershire sauce

1. Pat the steaks dry with paper towels and season with salt and pepper.

2. In a large cast iron skillet over medium-high heat, warm 1 tablespoon of olive oil for 5 minutes, or until the skillet is smoking. Add the steaks and cook for about 2 minutes on each side, until browned.

3. Reduce the temperature to medium and add the butter, letting it melt completely. Baste the steaks with the butter until your desired doneness is reached. Transfer the steaks to a platter and pour the butter over them. Let rest for 10 minutes.

4. In the same skillet over medium-high heat, add the remaining 1 tablespoon of olive oil and the garlic and cook until the garlic becomes fragrant. Add the mushrooms and onions and cook for about 8 minutes, until the onions are tender and browned. Add the Worcestershire sauce and cook for an additional 2 minutes. Season with salt and pepper.

5. Serve the steaks with the sautéed mushrooms and onions.

Per Serving: **Calories: 579; Total Fat: 49g; Protein: 28g; Total Carbohydrates: 6g; Fiber: 1g; Net Carbs: 5g**

Macros: **Fat: 76%; Protein: 19%; Carbs: 5%**

Beef Skewers with Balsamic-Soy Cabbage

SERVES

MARINATE TIME

PREP TIME

COOK TIME

This Asian-style beef reaches optimal flavor when marinated for at least 12 hours and can be made days in advance for convenience. It's a wonderful dish for a family get-together; they are quite simple to cook, and the kids will like the skewers. You will need long bamboo skewers for this recipe.

¾ cup extra-virgin olive oil, divided

¼ cup plus 1 tablespoon soy sauce

¼ cup plus 1 tablespoon balsamic vinegar

1 tablespoon Swerve brown sugar sweetener

2 tablespoons minced garlic cloves, divided

Salt

Freshly ground black pepper

1 (1½-pound) flank steak, cut into ¼-inch slices

4 cups shredded cabbage

1. In a large resealable bag, add ¼ cup of olive oil, ¼ cup of soy sauce, ¼ cup of balsamic vinegar, the Swerve, 1¾ tablespoons of garlic, salt, and pepper. Add the steak, seal the bag, and refrigerate for at least 2 (and up to 24) hours.

2. In a mixing bowl, mix together the remaining 1 tablespoon of soy sauce, 1 tablespoon of balsamic vinegar, 1 teaspoon of minced garlic, and ½ cup of olive oil and season with salt and pepper. Add the shredded cabbage and mix well to combine. Cover with plastic wrap and refrigerate until ready to serve.

3. Soak the skewers in water for 30 minutes.

4. Preheat a gas or charcoal grill to medium-high heat.

5. Thread each slice of flank steak onto an individual skewer. Grill for 2 to 3 minutes per side.

6. Serve alongside the balsamic-soy cabbage.

Substitution tip: Chicken breasts work well as a substitute for the flank steak.

Per Serving: Calories: 632; Total Fat: 50g; Protein: 39g; Total Carbohydrates: 7g; Fiber: 2g; Net Carbs: 5g; Sweetener Carbs: 2g

Macros: Fat: 71%; Protein: 25%; Carbs: 4%

Filet Mignon with Mushrooms and Sage Brown Butter

GLUTEN-FREE / ONE-POT

Sage is an herb that is loaded with antioxidants, and it brings a wonderful flavor to a strong stand-alone type of protein like filet mignon.

4 (5-ounce) filet mignon steaks, at room temperature

Salt

Freshly ground black pepper

2 tablespoons extra-virgin olive oil, divided

1 pound sliced mushrooms

½ medium onion, sliced

2 garlic cloves, chopped

4 tablespoons butter

6 fresh sage leaves

1. Season the steaks with salt and pepper.

2. In a skillet over medium-high heat, warm 1 tablespoon of olive oil. Add the steaks and cook on both sides to your desired temperature. Transfer the steaks to a plate and set aside.

3. Reduce the heat to medium and add the remaining 1 tablespoon of olive oil. Add the mushrooms and onions and cook for 5 to 7 minutes. Add the garlic and cook for 2 more minutes. Season with salt and pepper and transfer to the plate with the steaks.

4. Add the butter and sage leaves to the skillet and cook for 3 to 5 minutes, until the butter smells nutty and has browned. Remove the sage leaves and discard.

5. Serve the steaks with the mushrooms and onions and drizzle them with the sage brown butter.

Make it vegetarian: **Make this dish vegetarian by serving the mushrooms, onions, and sage brown butter over a bed of spaghetti squash and topped with toasted walnuts.**

Per Serving: **Calories: 420; Total Fat: 28g; Protein: 36g; Total Carbohydrates: 6g; Fiber: 2g; Net Carbs: 4g;**

Macros: **Fat: 60%; Protein: 34%; Carbs: 6%**

Skirt Steak and Broccoli Florets

DAIRY-FREE / ONE-POT

Marinate the meat on a Sunday, and you'll be able to serve this is meal on a busy Monday evening. I really love the sweet and salty flavors of the brown sugar and soy sauce.

SERVES

4

MARINATE TIME

PREP TIME

COOK TIME

⅓ cup plus 2 teaspoons soy sauce

¼ cup plus ½ teaspoon balsamic vinegar

3 tablespoons plus 1 teaspoon grated garlic, divided

1 tablespoon Swerve brown sugar sweetener

Salt

Freshly ground black pepper

1 (1½-pound) skirt steak

2 tablespoons extra-virgin olive oil, divided

6 cups 2-inch broccoli florets

1. Combine the soy sauce, balsamic vinegar, 3 tablespoons of garlic, and Swerve to a large resealable bag. Season with salt and pepper. Add the skirt steak, seal the bag, and refrigerate for at least 4 (and up to 24) hours.

2. Remove the steak from the marinade and let it sit at room temperature for about 20 minutes.

3. In a large skillet over medium-high heat, warm 1 tablespoon of olive oil. Add the skirt steak and cook for 3 to 5 minutes per side, until your desired temperature is reached. Transfer the steak to a plate and let it rest for at least 5 minutes.

4. In the same skillet, add the remaining 1 tablespoon of olive oil and the broccoli and sauté for 3 minutes. Add the remaining 1 teaspoon of garlic, 2 teaspoons of soy sauce, and ½ teaspoon of balsamic vinegar and sauté for about 3 minutes, until the broccoli is fork tender. Season with salt and pepper.

5. Carve the skirt steak crosswise into thin slices and serve alongside the broccoli.

Substitution tip: A flank steak or a flat-iron steak can be substituted for the skirt steak.

Per Serving: Calories: 425; Total Fat: 23g; Protein: 42g; Total Carbohydrates: 13g; Fiber: 4g; Net Carbs: 9g; Sweetener Carbs: 3g

Macros: Fat: 49%; Protein: 40%; Carbs: 11%

Red Wine Beef Short Ribs with Carrots and Parsnips

SERVES

4

PREP TIME

COOK TIME

DAIRY-FREE / ONE-POT

Nothing says comfort food more than a savory dish that has been cooking for hours and fills the home with amazing aromas. This meal will give you an excuse to gather family or friends around the kitchen table and enjoy a wonderful Sunday meal together. The carrots and parsnips can be served whole or mashed, which is what I prefer—mashed vegetables really up the comfort factor.

2 pounds beef short ribs

Salt

Freshly ground black pepper

2 tablespoons extra-virgin olive oil

2 tablespoons chopped garlic

3 carrots, peeled and quartered

3 parsnips, peeled and quartered

1 cup red wine

1 tablespoon tomato paste

½ cup water

1. Preheat the oven to 350°F.

2. Season the short ribs with salt and pepper.

3. In a large Dutch oven over medium-high heat, warm the olive oil. Add the garlic and cook until the garlic becomes fragrant. Add the short ribs to the skillet and cook for about 5 minutes per side, until they begin to brown. Transfer the ribs to a plate and set aside.

4. Add the carrots and parsnips to the Dutch oven and cook until they begin to brown. Add the red wine, tomato paste, water, and the short ribs along with any drippings. Season with salt and pepper.

5. Cover and bake for 2½ to 3 hours, or until the short ribs are fork tender.

Simplify it: This dish can also be cooked in a slow cooker. After step 3, add all of the ingredients to a slow cooker and cook on low for 6 to 8 hours.

Per Serving: Calories: 691; Total Fat: 47g; Protein: 42g; Total Carbohydrates: 25g; Fiber: 7g; Net Carbs: 18g

Macros: Fat: 61%; Protein: 24%; Carbs: 15%

Veal Meatballs with Roasted Tomatoes

GLUTEN-FREE / ONE-PAN

SERVES

4

PREP
TIME

20

COOK
TIME

20

Meatballs are always a winner in my house. I like to make a big batch of these and freeze them individually, which makes it easy to take out as many as I need during the week. You can also substitute ground beef for the veal.

4 cups grape tomatoes

¾ tablespoon grated garlic, divided

1 tablespoon extra-virgin olive oil

½ teaspoon salt, divided

1 teaspoon freshly ground black pepper, divided

1 pound ground veal

1 cup grated Parmesan cheese, divided

1 large egg

1 tablespoon Italian seasoning

1. Preheat the oven to 400°F. Line a baking sheet with parchment paper.

2. In a mixing bowl, mix together the grape tomatoes, ½ tablespoon of garlic, olive oil, ¼ teaspoon of salt, and ½ teaspoon of pepper and place on one side of the baking sheet.

3. In the same bowl, mix together the ground veal, ¾ cup of Parmesan cheese, egg, Italian seasoning, remaining ¼ tablespoon of garlic, ¼ teaspoon of salt, and ½ teaspoon of pepper. Form the mixture into 12 meatballs and place them on the baking sheet.

4. Roast for 20 minutes, turning the meatballs halfway through, until their internal temperature reaches 165°F.

5. Preheat the broiler. Sprinkle the remaining Parmesan cheese over the top of the meatballs and place them under the broiler until browned.

6. Serve the meatballs atop the roasted tomatoes.

Per Serving: **Calories: 384; Total Fat: 24g; Protein: 33g; Total Carbohydrates: 9g; Fiber: 2g; Net Carbs: 7g**

Macros: **Fat: 56%; Protein: 34%; Carbs: 10%**

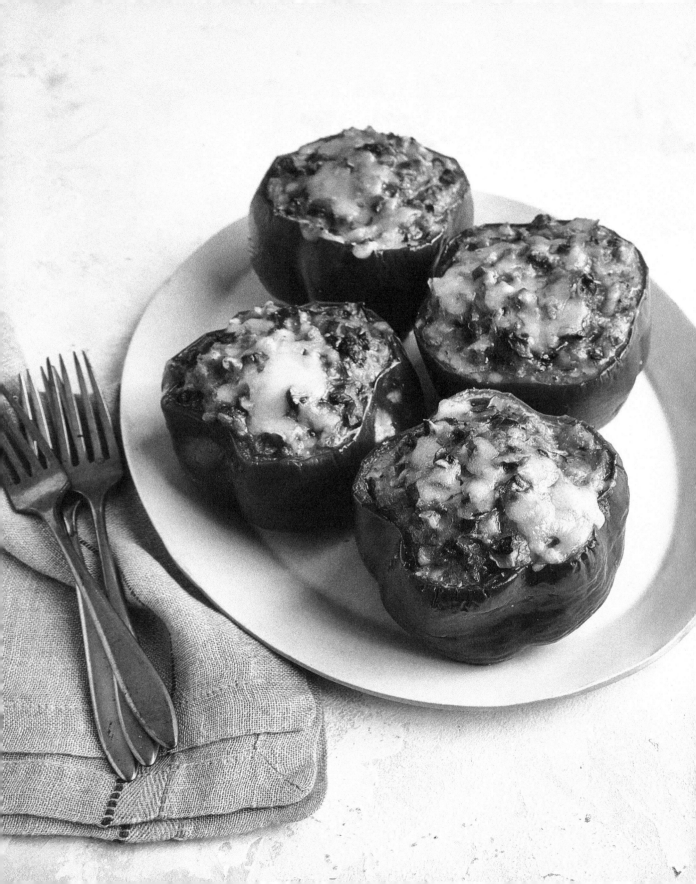

7.

Vegetarian Mains

< Cajun Stuffed Bell Peppers, *page 108*

Chili Roasted Tofu and Vegetables

SERVES

4

PREP
TIME

10

COOK
TIME

20

30-MINUTE / GLUTEN-FREE / VEGAN

Tofu is a soy-based protein that is rich in iron, calcium, and omega-3 fatty acids. Paired together with bell peppers and the superfood kale, this meal is a nutritious and well-balanced winner.

16 ounces firm tofu, cut into cubes

2 cups sliced red bell peppers

1 red onion, sliced

2 cups chopped kale

8 garlic cloves, peeled and halved

2 tablespoons chili powder

Salt

Freshly ground black pepper

Extra-virgin olive oil, for drizzling

1. Preheat the oven to 400°F. Line a baking sheet with parchment paper.

2. Place the tofu, bell peppers, red onion, and kale on the prepared baking sheet. Add the garlic, chili powder, salt, and pepper and toss. Drizzle with olive oil and mix all of the ingredients well.

3. Bake for 20 minutes, or until the tofu begins to brown and the vegetables are tender.

Substitution tip: **Not a fan of tofu? Use mushrooms instead.**

Per Serving: **Calories: 170; Total Fat: 6g; Protein: 12g; Total Carbohydrates: 17g; Fiber: 4g; Net Carbs: 13g**

Macros: **Fat: 32%; Protein: 28%; Carbs: 40%**

Bella Mushrooms with Red Pepper Sauce

GLUTEN-FREE / VEGAN

SERVES

4

PREP TIME

15

COOK TIME

45

I have learned that cashews are quite magical when it comes to vegan cooking because they can add creaminess without adding dairy. They serve as the creamy base in this low-carb recipe and, combined with the flavors of the roasted red peppers and garlic, they create a sauce that is quite amazing.

1 cup raw cashews

2 large red bell peppers

2 garlic cloves, peeled

4 tablespoons extra-virgin olive oil, divided

¼ cup fresh basil, plus more for garnish

3 tablespoons hot water

1½ teaspoons salt, divided

1 teaspoon freshly ground black pepper, divided

4 large portobello mushrooms, stems removed, gills removed, and thinly sliced

10 ounces fresh baby spinach

1. Preheat the oven to 400°F. Line a baking sheet with parchment paper.

2. Place the cashews in a bowl and cover them completely with water. Let them soak for at least 30 minutes.

3. Place the bell peppers and garlic cloves on the prepared baking sheet. Drizzle with 2 tablespoons of olive oil and bake for 30 minutes, turning the peppers every 10 minutes to prevent burning.

4. Place the bell peppers in a covered bowl and let them sit for 10 minutes. Remove the skin, seeds, and stems.

5. Drain the cashews. Add the bell peppers, roasted garlic, cashews, basil, 1 tablespoon of olive oil, and hot water to a blender and puree until creamy. Season with ½ teaspoon of salt and ½ teaspoon of black pepper. If the sauce is a bit thick, blend with a little more hot water until you reach your desired consistency.

Continued >

6. In a large skillet over medium-high heat, warm the remaining 1 tablespoon of olive oil for 30 seconds. Add the mushrooms and cook for about 3 minutes. Add the baby spinach and cook for 2 to 3 minutes, until the spinach is slightly wilted. Season with the remaining salt and pepper.

7. Divide the vegetables between 4 shallow bowls and spoon the roasted red pepper sauce over the top. Garnish with more basil.

Substitution tip: **You can substitute zucchini noodles for the mushrooms. Add the zucchini to the skillet when the spinach is just wilted, turn off the heat, cover, and allow it to sit for about 3 minutes. You want the zucchini to be al dente.**

Per Serving: **Calories: 344; Total Fat: 24g; Protein: 12g; Total Carbohydrates: 20g; Fiber: 5g; Net Carbs: 15g**

Macros: **Fat: 63%; Protein: 14%; Carbs: 23%**

Greek Stuffed Eggplant

GLUTEN-FREE / VEGETARIAN

Greek cuisine is very flavorful and full of heart-healthy fats, often from plant-based ingredients. This recipe definitely meets those standards. Roasted eggplant combined with artichokes, olives, salty cheese, and freshly squeezed lemon juice offer the perfect, bold, low-carb combination.

2 medium eggplants, each cut in half lengthwise

3 tablespoons extra-virgin olive oil, divided

Salt

Freshly ground black pepper

1½ cups riced cauliflower

2 garlic cloves, chopped

½ cup chopped artichoke hearts

½ cup sliced Greek olives

Juice of ½ lemon

1½ cups grated Parmesan cheese

1. Preheat the oven to 400°F. Line a baking sheet with parchment paper.

2. Score the eggplant on the cut side in a crosshatch pattern about ½ inch deep. Drizzle with 2 tablespoons of olive oil and season with salt and pepper.

3. Bake for 30 minutes, or until it becomes browned and fork tender. Using a spoon, scoop about ¼ of the pulp from each eggplant half, roughly chop it, and set it aside. Place the eggplant shells on the prepared baking sheet.

4. In a skillet over medium-high heat, warm the remaining 1 tablespoon of olive oil. Add the riced cauliflower and garlic and cook for 5 minutes. Add the chopped eggplant, artichoke hearts, olives, and lemon juice and cook for an additional 2 minutes. Season with salt and pepper.

5. Set the oven to broil. Divide the mixture equally between the eggplant shells. Sprinkle the tops with the Parmesan cheese. Broil until the cheese is melted and slightly browned.

Per Serving: **Calories: 286; Total Fat: 18g; Protein: 9g; Total Carbohydrates: 22g; Fiber: 12g; Net Carbs: 10g**

Macros: **Fat: 57%; Protein: 12%; Carbs: 31%**

Puttanesca with Sautéed Kale

30-MINUTE / GLUTEN-FREE / ONE-POT / VEGAN

SERVES

4

PREP
TIME

10

COOK
TIME

15

Puttanesca is an Italian pasta dish from Naples that includes anchovies and capers, which give it a salty and briny flavor. A sheet of nori seaweed serves as the perfect substitute for the anchovies here, making this a vegan crowd-pleaser.

1 sheet nori

1 tablespoon extra-virgin olive oil

3 garlic cloves, chopped

16 ounces shredded kale

½ cup kalamata olives, plus 1 teaspoon brine

2 cups diced fresh tomatoes

¼ cup capers, plus 1 teaspoon brine

Salt

Freshly ground black pepper

1. Place the nori sheet in a blender and blend until it becomes a powder.

2. In a large skillet over medium-high heat, warm the olive oil. Add the garlic and cook until it becomes fragrant. Add the kale and sauté for 5 minutes.

3. Add the olives, olive brine, ground nori, tomatoes, capers, and the caper brine. Cook for an additional 3 to 5 minutes. Season with salt and pepper and serve.

Simplify it: **Canned diced or crushed tomatoes will work well in place of the fresh tomatoes.**

Per Serving: **Calories: 146; Total Fat: 6g; Protein: 5g; Total Carbohydrates: 18g; Fiber: 4g; Net Carbs: 14g**

Macros: **Fat: 37%; Protein: 14%; Carbs: 49%**

Cauliflower Steak Pizzas

GLUTEN-FREE / ONE-POT / VEGETARIAN

Who says you can't eat pizza on a low-carb diet? This healthy version will make you never miss your old pizza pie. Roasted cauliflower steaks make an incredible base for a medley of vitamin-rich vegetables that bring crunch and flavor to the party.

SERVES

4

PREP TIME

10

COOK TIME

30

4 (1-inch-thick) cauliflower steaks

2 garlic cloves, chopped

Salt

Freshly ground black pepper

2 tablespoons extra-virgin olive oil

¼ cup canned crushed tomatoes

1 cup fresh baby spinach

1 red bell pepper, thinly sliced

¼ cup shredded mozzarella cheese

1. Preheat the oven to 400°F. Line a baking sheet with parchment paper.

2. Season both sides of the cauliflower steaks with the garlic, salt, pepper, and olive oil. Bake for 15 minutes, turn them over, and cook for another 10 minutes.

3. Set the oven to broil. Add the tomatoes to the steaks and season with salt and pepper. Top with the baby spinach, bell pepper, and mozzarella cheese.

4. Broil the pizzas, until the cheese is browed and bubbly.

Make it vegan: Replace the mozzarella with a vegan cheese or a dollop of dairy-free pesto.

Per Serving: **Calories: 157; Total Fat: 9g; Protein: 6g; Total Carbohydrates: 13g; Fiber: 5g; Net Carbs: 8g**

Macros: **Fat: 52%; Protein: 33%; Carbs: 15%**

Cajun Stuffed Bell Peppers

GLUTEN-FREE / VEGETARIAN

SERVES

4

PREP
TIME

10

COOK
TIME

35

Cajun stuffed peppers make for a wonderful, easy meal. Traditionally made with andouille sausage and rice, this low-carb vegetarian version is nutritious, flavorful, and quite filling.

4 green bell peppers, tops removed and chopped, seeded, and reserved

1 tablespoon extra-virgin olive oil

4 garlic cloves, chopped

4 cups chopped mushrooms

2 cups riced cauliflower

2 tablespoons Cajun Seasoning (see page 131)

1 teaspoon salt

1 teaspoon freshly ground black pepper

1 cup shredded pepper jack cheese

1. Preheat the oven to 400°F. Have a baking dish ready.

2. Place the bell pepper shells in the baking dish.

3. In a skillet over medium-high heat, warm the olive oil. Add the garlic and cook until it becomes fragrant. Add the mushrooms, cauliflower, chopped bell pepper tops, and the Cajun seasoning and cook for 8 to 10 minutes. Season with salt and pepper. Remove from the heat and allow to cool for 10 minutes.

4. Add the pepper jack cheese to the mixture and mix well.

5. Fill each bell pepper with the vegetable and cheese mixture and bake for 15 to 20 minutes, or until the peppers are browned and the cheese is melted.

Variation: **Make this an Italian dish by replacing the Cajun seasoning with your favorite Italian seasoning blend and using mozzarella instead of pepper jack cheese. Make this a Greek dish by replacing the seasoning with a Greek blend and using feta instead of pepper jack.**

Per Serving: **Calories: 213; Total Fat: 13g; Protein: 12g; Total Carbohydrates: 12g; Fiber: 4g; Net Carbs: 8g**

Macros: **Fat: 54%; Protein: 23%; Carbs: 23%**

Southwest Spaghetti Squash

Adding avocado to any recipe is almost always a wonderful idea. It offers many health benefits: Avocados are heart-healthy, high in fiber, and provide more potassium than a banana. Combined with the vegetables in this dish, you have a well-balanced, low-carb dish.

SERVES

4

PREP TIME

5

COOK TIME

50

2 (2- to 2½-pound) spaghetti squash, cut in half lengthwise

3 teaspoons salt, divided

1½ teaspoons freshly ground black pepper, divided

4 tablespoons extra-virgin olive oil, divided

3 garlic cloves, chopped

16 ounces zucchini, chopped

1 tablespoon ground cumin

½ cup pico de gallo

2 avocados, diced

1. Preheat the oven to 400°F. Line a baking sheet with parchment paper.

2. Scoop out the seeds of the spaghetti squash. Season the inside with 2 teaspoons of salt and 1 teaspoon of pepper and rub with 2 tablespoons of olive oil.

3. Place the spaghetti squash, cut-side down, on the prepared baking sheet and roast for 30 to 40 minutes, or until the meat is fork tender. Let cool.

4. When cool to the touch, cut each squash into halves, crosswise, and loosen the strands with a fork. Drizzle with 1 tablespoon of olive oil.

5. In a skillet over medium-high heat, warm the remaining 1 tablespoon of olive oil. Add the garlic and cook until it becomes fragrant. Add the zucchini and cumin and cook for about 5 minutes, until the zucchini begins to brown. Season with the remaining 1 teaspoon of salt and ½ teaspoon of pepper and cook for an additional 2 minutes.

6. Spoon the zucchini into the squash bowls and top with pico de gallo and avocado.

Per Serving: Calories: 410; Total Fat: 30g; Protein: 5g; Total Carbohydrates: 30g; Fiber: 8g; Net Carbs: 22g

Macros: Fat: 66%; Protein: 5%; Carbs: 29%

Zoodle Primavera with Toasted Walnuts

SERVES

4

PREP
TIME

20

COOK
TIME

10

30-MINUTE / GLUTEN-FREE / ONE-POT / VEGAN

Toasted walnuts are really the star in this recipe. In the culinary world, they are often referred to as "brain food." It has been suggested that consuming them on a consistent basis aids in better brain function. They are even known to help lower cholesterol, too.

2 tablespoons extra-virgin olive oil, divided

2 cups quartered mushrooms

¼ cup walnut halves

2 garlic cloves, chopped

3 zucchinis, spiralized or cut into ribbons

2 cups thinly sliced red bell peppers

¼ cup thinly sliced fresh basil

Salt

Freshly ground black pepper

1. In a skillet over medium-high heat, warm 1 tablespoon of olive oil. Add the mushrooms and cook for about 3 minutes, until they begin to brown. Add the walnuts and garlic and cook for an additional 2 to 3 minutes, stirring often.

2. Add the zucchini and bell peppers. Cook for about 2 minutes, just enough to warm the zucchini without it becoming mushy. Add the remaining 1 tablespoon of olive oil and the basil and mix well. Season with salt and pepper.

Variation: Swap the basil and walnuts out for pesto and a splash of half-and-half to make a richer, creamier sauce.

Per Serving: Calories: 154; Total Fat: 10g; Protein: 4g; Total Carbohydrates: 12g; Fiber: 3g; Net Carbs: 9g

Macros: Fat: 58%; Protein: 11%; Carbs: 31%

Edamame Bowls

30-MINUTE / GLUTEN-FREE / ONE-POT / VEGAN

Edamame is a soybean, rich in antioxidants and fiber. Sautéing the edamame with the bell peppers and cabbage transforms these already flavorful ingredients into an even-tastier combo, bringing out the subtle sweetness of the vegetables. Finish with freshly squeezed lemon juice to bring a pop of sunshine to the dish.

SERVES

PREP
TIME

COOK
TIME

1 tablespoon extra-virgin olive oil

4 garlic cloves, chopped

2 teaspoons grated fresh ginger

1 pound shelled edamame

1 large red bell pepper, chopped

1 cup chopped red cabbage

Juice of ½ lemon

Salt

Freshly ground black pepper

¼ cup chopped roasted almonds

1. In a large skillet over medium-high heat, warm the olive oil. Add the garlic and ginger and cook for 30 seconds. Add the edamame, bell peppers, and cabbage and sauté for 6 to 8 minutes, until the vegetables are tender. Add the lemon juice and season with salt and pepper.

2. Garnish each bowl with the chopped roasted almonds.

Variation: **Remove the ginger and add basil, thyme, rosemary, or dill instead.**

Per Serving: **Calories: 241; Total Fat: 13g; Protein: 14g; Total Carbohydrates: 17g; Fiber: 5g; Net Carbs: 12g**

Macros: **Fat: 49%; Protein: 23%; Carbs: 28%**

Collard Green Egg Salad Wraps

30-MINUTE / GLUTEN-FREE / VEGETARIAN

SERVES

4

PREP
TIME

10

COOK
TIME

8

Egg salad is one of my favorite low-carb meals because it is so versatile and forgiving. You seriously cannot go wrong with anything you add to the mix. In this recipe, I've added curry powder for a lovely kick. When this egg salad is swaddled in a collard greens wrap, which is high in vitamin C, iron, and fiber, you have a handheld, nutritious meal that only takes minutes to prepare.

8 large eggs

⅓ cup mayonnaise

1 teaspoon curry powder

1 teaspoon freshly squeezed lemon juice

½ teaspoon salt

½ teaspoon freshly ground black pepper

4 large collard greens leaves, stems removed

1 cup alfalfa sprouts

1. Place the eggs in a large saucepan and cover with cold water by 1 inch. Slowly bring water to a boil over medium heat, cover, and turn off the heat. Let the eggs sit for 8 minutes. Drain the water and gently crack the eggs while running under cold water. Chop the eggs into small pieces and set aside.

2. In a mixing bowl, combine the eggs, mayonnaise, curry powder, lemon juice, salt, and pepper.

3. Divide the egg salad between the 4 collard greens leaves. Top with alfalfa sprouts and roll the wrap like a burrito.

Variation: **Instead of curry powder, try this dish with my Cajun Seasoning (see page 131) for an even bolder flavor profile.**

Per Serving: **Calories: 309; Total Fat: 25g; Protein: 14g; Total Carbohydrates: 7g; Fiber: 4g; Net Carbs: 3g**

Macros: **Fat: 73%; Protein: 18%; Carbs: 9%**

Cabbage Steaks with Vegetables and Blue Cheese

30-MINUTE / GLUTEN-FREE / VEGETARIAN

SERVES

4

PREP TIME

10

COOK TIME

20

This recipe is a cross between nachos and a stacked protein casserole. Cabbage makes an ideal base to stack your favorite ingredients. The small amount of balsamic vinegar really rounds this dish out.

1 head cabbage, cut into ½-inch slices

Salt

Freshly ground black pepper

1 tablespoon extra-virgin olive oil, plus more for drizzling

2 garlic cloves, chopped

24 spears asparagus, cut into bite-size pieces

1 cup halved grape tomatoes

¼ cup crumbled blue cheese

2 tablespoons balsamic vinegar

1. Preheat a gas or charcoal grill to medium-high. Have a baking sheet ready.

2. Season both sides of the cabbage steaks with salt and pepper. Drizzle with olive oil and set aside.

3. In a skillet over medium-high heat, warm 1 tablespoon of olive oil. Add the garlic and cook for about 30 seconds, until fragrant. Add the asparagus and sauté for about 5 minutes, until tender.

4. Grill the cabbage steaks for about 5 minutes per side. Transfer the steaks to the baking sheet. Top each steak with the tomatoes, asparagus, blue cheese crumbles, and balsamic vinegar. Season with salt and pepper.

5. Close the lid on the grill and cook for an additional 5 to 7 minutes, or until the cheese is melted and the tomatoes begin to slightly cook.

Substitution tip: Instead of cabbage steaks, you can use cauliflower steaks from my Chicken and Cauliflower Steaks Provolone (see page 77).

Per Serving: Calories: 154; Total Fat: 6g; Protein: 8g; Total Carbohydrates: 17g; Fiber: 9g; Net Carbs: 8g

Macros: Fat: 35%; Protein: 21%; Carbs: 44%

Artichoke-Stuffed Mushrooms

GLUTEN-FREE / VEGETARIAN

SERVES

4

PREP
TIME

10

COOK
TIME

25

For this recipe, I took my favorite spinach-artichoke dip and transformed it into a low-carb meal that has fewer calories and less fat. It provides a delicious blend of vegetables and cheese, contrasted by the crunch of roasted almonds.

4 large portobello mushrooms, gills removed and discarded, stems chopped and reserved

2 teaspoons salt, divided

1 teaspoon freshly ground black pepper, divided

2 tablespoons extra-virgin olive oil, divided

3 garlic cloves, chopped

8 cups fresh spinach

14 ounces artichoke hearts, roughly chopped

1 cup grated Parmesan cheese

¼ cup chopped roasted almonds

1. Preheat the oven to 400°F. Line a baking sheet with parchment paper.

2. Season both sides of the mushrooms with 1 teaspoon of salt and ½ teaspoon of pepper.

3. In a skillet over medium-high heat, warm 1 tablespoon of olive oil for 30 seconds. Add the mushroom caps and cook for 1 to 2 minutes on each side, until slightly browned. Transfer to a plate and cover with an inverted bowl to allow the liquid to drain.

4. In the same skillet, warm the remaining 1 tablespoon of olive oil. Add the garlic and cook until it becomes fragrant. Add the spinach, artichoke hearts, and chopped mushroom stems and cook for about 5 minutes, until the spinach begins to wilt. Remove from the heat and let cool for 5 minutes.

5. Add the Parmesan cheese and mix well to incorporate. Season with the remaining salt and pepper.

6. Place the mushroom caps on the prepared baking sheet. Spoon the vegetable mixture equally into the mushroom caps and top each with crushed almonds. Bake for 10 to 15 minutes, or until they become lightly browned.

Per Serving: **Calories: 292; Total Fat: 16g; Protein: 18g; Total Carbohydrates: 19g; Fiber: 9g; Net Carbs: 10g**

Macros: **Fat: 49%; Protein: 25%; Carbs: 26%**

Zucchini and Squash Tomato Gratin

GLUTEN-FREE / VEGETARIAN

This decadent dish is a favorite at potlucks and picnics across the South, where vegetables and cheese are both important food groups!

1 tablespoon extra-virgin olive oil, plus more for greasing

2 garlic cloves, chopped

2 zucchinis, diced

2 yellow squash, diced

1 large egg

1 teaspoon salt

½ teaspoon freshly ground black pepper

2 Roma tomatoes, thinly sliced

2 ounces Gruyère cheese, shredded

1. Preheat the oven to 350°F. Grease an 8-by-8-inch baking dish.

2. In a large skillet over medium-high heat, warm the olive oil. Add the garlic and cook until it becomes fragrant. Add the zucchini and yellow squash and cook until the vegetables become browned and tender, about 6 minutes.

3. Using a fork, roughly mash the vegetables, leaving some chunky pieces. Transfer to a colander to drain any excess liquid.

4. In a mixing bowl, mix together the zucchini-squash mixture, egg, salt, and pepper.

5. Arrange a layer of the sliced tomatoes on the bottom of the baking dish. Spread the squash mixture over the bottom layer of tomatoes, and then top with the remaining tomato slices.

6. Bake for 10 minutes. Sprinkle the Gruyère cheese over the top and bake for an additional 20 minutes, until the cheese is melted and begins to brown.

Substitution tip: **Swiss cheese would be an ideal substitution for the Gruyère cheese.**

Per Serving: **Calories: 153; Total Fat: 9g; Protein: 8g; Total Carbohydrates: 10g; Fiber: 3g; Net Carbs: 7g**

Macros: **Fat: 53%; Protein: 21%; Carbs: 26%**

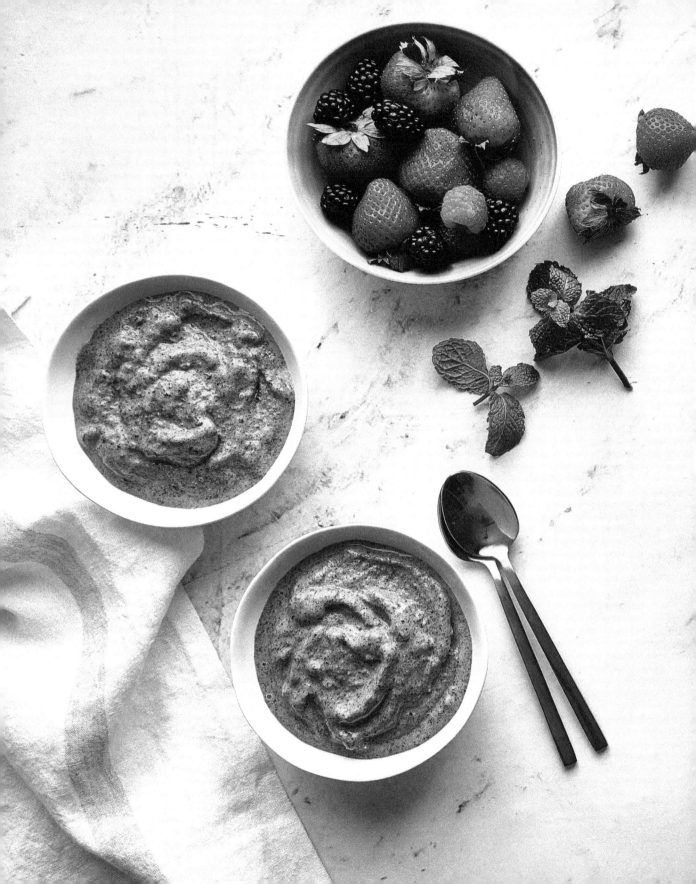

8.

Desserts, Dressings, and Staples

< Mixed Berry and Lime Sorbet, *page 118*

Mixed Berry and Lime Sorbet

30-MINUTE / GLUTEN-FREE / ONE-POT / VEGAN

SERVES

4

PREP
TIME

15

This is the easiest dessert you will ever make. It goes from frozen berries to sorbet to your mouth in minutes. The lime adds a subtle tartness against the sweetness of the Swerve.

16 ounces frozen berries

Juice of ½ lime

1 teaspoon Swerve granulated sweetener

¼ cup half-and-half

½ teaspoon salt

1 to 2 tablespoons warm water

In a food processor, process the berries, lime juice, Swerve, half-and-half, and salt, stopping often to scrape down the sides. Add the warm water in intervals to help smooth out the berries. Serve immediately.

Simplify it: **Read the label on the frozen berries. There shouldn't be any ingredients except fruit.**

Per Serving: **Calories: 82; Total Fat: 2g; Protein: 1g; Total Carbohydrates: 15g; Fiber: 4g; Net Carbs: 11g; Sweetener Carbs: 1g**

Macros: **Fat: 22%; Protein: 5%; Carbs: 73%**

Almond Butter Cookie Dough Dip

30-MINUTE / GLUTEN-FREE / ONE-POT / VEGETARIAN

SERVES

PREP
TIME

Let me introduce you to almond butter cookie dough dip. Dunk a fresh strawberry into this sweet treat or eat it with a spoon for a low-carb indulgence that you will always want to keep stocked in your refrigerator.

8 ounces cream cheese, softened

½ cup almond butter

¼ cup Swerve granulated sweetener

1 teaspoon vanilla extract

¼ teaspoon salt

¼ cup sugar-free chocolate chips

1. In a mixing bowl, mix together the cream cheese, almond butter, Swerve, vanilla extract, and salt until creamy.

2. Fold in the chocolate chips.

Variations: **Swap the almond butter for peanut butter, cashew butter, or your favorite nut butter and the chocolate chips for your favorite berry.**

Per Serving: **Calories: 439; Total Fat: 38g; Protein: 9g; Total Carbohydrates: 15g; Fiber: 2g; Net Carbs: 13g; Sweetener Carbs: 12g**

Macros: **Fat: 78%; Protein: 8%; Carbs: 14%**

Avocado Chocolate Pudding

30-MINUTE / GLUTEN-FREE / ONE-POT / VEGAN

SERVES

PREP
TIME

The glorious avocado, with its healthy fat and large amount of fiber, also brings incredible creaminess to the plate in this sweet and healthy dessert. Offset by the rich cocoa powder, this pudding is a showstopper. I have been known to eat this pudding for breakfast!

3 avocados, pitted
and peeled

¾ cup unsweetened
almond milk

6 tablespoons
cocoa powder

¼ cup Swerve granulated
sweetener

2 teaspoons
vanilla extract

¼ teaspoon salt

In a food processor or blender, purée the avocados, almond milk, cocoa powder, sweetener, vanilla, and salt until smooth and creamy. Depending on the size of the avocados, you may need to adjust the amount of almond milk.

Variation: Substitute the cocoa out for your favorite low-carb powdered peanut butter.

Per Serving: Calories: 282; Total Fat: 22g; Protein: 5g; Total Carbohydrates: 16g; Fiber: 12g; Net Carbs: 4g; Sweetener Carbs: 12g

Macros: Fat: 70%; Protein: 7%; Carbs: 23%

Fudge with Pecans

30-MINUTE / GLUTEN-FREE / ONE-POT / VEGETARIAN

Keep this easy, low-carb fudge in the refrigerator for when those cravings for sweets hit. With only four ingredients, this fudge will definitely be a winner in your house. It also makes a wonderful hostess gift.

SERVES

4

PREP TIME

COOK TIME

16 ounces sugar-free chocolate chips

½ cup heavy whipping cream

¼ cup Swerve confectioners' sweetener

½ cup chopped pecans

1. Line an 8-by-8-inch baking dish with parchment paper.

2. In a microwave safe bowl, mix together the chocolate chips, heavy whipping cream, and Swerve. Microwave on high for 1 minute and stir. Continue to microwave in 20 second intervals, stirring in between, until the chocolate is completely melted and the ingredients are combined. Stir in the pecans.

3. Spread the mixture out in the prepared baking dish and let it cool. Cut into squares and serve.

Variation: **Swap out the chocolate chips and pecans for white chocolate and peanuts.**

Per Serving: **Calories: 826; Total Fat: 70g; Protein: 17g; Total Carbohydrates: 32g; Fiber: 20g; Net Carbs: 12g; Sweetener Carbs: 12g**

Macros: **Fat: 76%; Protein: 9%; Carbs: 15%**

Lemon Cakes

30-MINUTE / GLUTEN-FREE / ONE-POT / VEGETARIAN

SERVES

4

PREP
TIME

5

COOK
TIME

2

Lemon is my favorite flavor in a dessert, and these speedy-to-make individual cakes allow me to partake in my favorite treat anytime I want.

Nonstick cooking spray or butter, for greasing

1½ cups almond flour

¼ cup Swerve confectioners' sweetener

2 teaspoons baking powder

1 teaspoon salt

½ cup freshly squeezed lemon juice

¼ cup coconut oil, melted

4 large eggs

1 tablespoon lemon zest

1. Lightly grease 4 microwave-safe mugs.

2. In a mixing bowl, mix together the almond flour, Swerve, baking powder, and salt. Add the lemon juice, coconut oil, eggs, and lemon zest and stir until combined.

3. Divide the batter equally between the 4 mugs. Microwave on high for 1½ minutes, or until cooked throughout.

Variation: **Try using an orange in place of the lemon for a bright and vibrant flavor.**

Per Serving: **Calories: 340; Total Fat: 30g; Protein: 11g; Total Carbohydrates: 8g; Fiber: 3g; Net Carbs: 5g; Sweetener Carbs: 12g**

Macros: **Fat: 79%; Protein: 13%; Carbs: 8%**

Pumpkin Pie Custard Bites

30-MINUTE / GLUTEN-FREE / ONE-POT / VEGETARIAN

Pumpkin is loaded with fiber and vitamin A, which is wonderful for heart health. So, there's no need for eater's remorse when eating this dessert—even if you eat it for breakfast. These bites are best eaten chilled and with a spoon.

MAKES

6

PREP TIME

10

COOK TIME

20

8 ounces cream cheese, softened

1 large egg, at room temperature

¼ cup pure pumpkin purée

¼ cup Swerve brown sugar sweetener

½ tablespoon pumpkin pie spice

¼ teaspoon salt

1. Preheat the oven to 350°F. Prepare a 6-cup muffin tin with paper or silicone liners.

2. In a mixing bowl, mix together the cream cheese and egg until smooth. Add the pumpkin purée, Swerve, pumpkin pie spice, and salt and mix until combined. Divide the batter equally between the muffin cups.

3. Bake for 20 minutes, or until the center is slightly firm and not completely set.

4. Let cool for 30 minutes and refrigerate until cold. Serve chilled.

Variation: **Replace the pumpkin pie purée and pumpkin pie spice with your favorite nut butter and ground cinnamon.**

Per Serving: **Calories: 149; Total Fat: 14g; Protein: 4g; Total Carbohydrates: 2g; Fiber: 0g; Net Carbs: 2g; Protein: 4g; Sweetener Carbs: 8g**

Macros: **Fat: 85%; Protein: 11%; Carbs: 4%**

Chocolate–Peanut Butter Mug Cakes

30-MINUTE / GLUTEN-FREE / ONE-POT / VEGETARIAN

The combination of chocolate and peanut butter reminds me of one of my favorite childhood candies. Think of this mug cake as a healthy adult version of those famous chocolate-covered peanut butter cups.

Nonstick cooking spray

½ cup peanut butter

½ cup Swerve brown sugar sweetener

½ teaspoon baking powder

4 eggs

¼ cup sugar-free dark chocolate chips

1. Spray 4 microwave-safe mugs with nonstick cooking spray.

2. In a small bowl, mix together the peanut butter, Swerve, baking powder, and eggs. Gently stir in the chocolate chips. Divide the mixture equally between the 4 mugs.

3. Microwave each mug for 1 minute and allow to rest for about 2 minutes.

Variations: **Use almond butter, cashew butter, or any other nut butter instead of peanut butter. You can also use chopped nuts instead of chocolate chips.**

Per Serving: **Calories: 325; Total Fat: 25g; Protein: 15g; Total Carbohydrates: 10g; Fiber: 3g; Net Carbs: 7g; Sweetener Carbs: 24g**

Macros: **Fat: 69%; Protein: 18%; Carbs: 13%**

Caramel Nuts and Whipped Cream

30-MINUTE / GLUTEN-FREE / VEGETARIAN

SERVES

4

PREP
TIME

5

COOK
TIME

15

Keep these ingredients in your pantry and refrigerator because you're going to want to make this all the time. And once you make homemade sugar-free whipped cream, you'll never buy it at the store again—it's that good.

4 tablespoons butter, divided

1 cup chopped pecans

1 cup chopped almonds

½ cup Swerve brown sugar sweetener

½ teaspoon salt

1 cup heavy whipping cream

1. Preheat the oven to 350°F. Line a baking sheet with parchment paper.

2. In a large skillet over medium-high heat, melt 2 tablespoons of butter. Add the pecans and almonds and toast for 1 minute. Transfer the nuts to a plate and set aside.

3. Reduce the heat to medium and melt the remaining butter. Add the Swerve and cook until the sugar dissolves. Add the nuts to the mixture and mix to coat evenly.

4. Transfer the nuts to the prepared baking sheet, sprinkle with the salt, and bake for 10 minutes. Let cool and break up any large pieces.

5. In the bowl of a stand mixer fitted with the whisk attachment, whip the heavy whipping cream on high until it forms stiff peaks.

6. Serve the candied nuts and whipped cream mixed together in bowls.

Per Serving: **Calories: 648; Total Fat: 63g; Protein: 10g; Total Carbohydrates: 11g; Fiber: 6g; Net Carbs: 5g; Sweetener Carbs: 24g**

Macros: **Fat: 88%; Protein: 6%; Carbs: 6%**

Ranch Dressing

SERVES

4

PREP TIME

10

This dressing is a staple and it's versatile, so you can alter the herbs to meet your specific recipe needs. Use it on salads, chicken, or as a marinade for your favorite fish.

½ cup half-and-half

½ cup mayonnaise

¼ cup sour cream

1 teaspoon dried dill

½ teaspoon grated garlic

½ teaspoon onion powder

Salt

Freshly ground black pepper

In a mixing bowl, mix together the half-and-half, mayonnaise, sour cream, dill, garlic, onion powder, salt, and pepper until smooth and creamy. Refrigerate until ready to serve.

Variation: Easily transform this dressing into jalapeño ranch by using pickled jalapeño juice in place of the half-and-half and substituting minced jalapeños in place of the dill.

Per Serving: Calories: 260; Total Fat: 27g; Protein: 2g; Total Carbohydrates: 2g; Fiber: 0g; Net Carbs: 2g;

Macros: Fat: 92%; Protein: 4%; Carbs: 4%

Avocado-Basil Dressing

30-MINUTE / GLUTEN-FREE / ONE-POT / VEGETARIAN

Here is a healthy, low-carb dressing that pairs well with fish, chicken, or a fresh garden salad. The avocado, basil, and lemon are what give this dressing its spunk!

SERVES

PREP TIME

½ cup half-and-half

¼ cup sour cream

¼ avocado

2 tablespoons chopped fresh basil

2 tablespoons mayonnaise

Juice of 1½ lemons

1 garlic clove, peeled

Salt

Freshly ground black pepper

In a blender, purée the half-and-half, sour cream, avocado, basil, mayonnaise, lemon juice, garlic, salt, and pepper until smooth and creamy. Season with salt and pepper.

Variation: Swap the lemon and basil out for lime and fresh dill.

Per Serving: Calories: 157; Total Fat: 15g; Protein: 2g; Total Carbohydrates: 4g; Fiber: 2g; Net Carbs: 2g

Macros: Fat: 86%; Protein: 5%; Carbs: 9%

Spinach-Basil Pesto

30-MINUTE / GLUTEN-FREE / ONE-POT / VEGETARIAN

SERVES

PREP
TIME

By adding spinach to this recipe, I've given traditional pesto a little twist. Pesto is a staple in my kitchen, and I use it all the time because it can transform a "blah" dish into something delicious.

2 cups fresh baby spinach

3 cups fresh basil

½ cup grated Parmesan cheese

½ cup walnut pieces

3 garlic cloves, peeled

Juice of 1 lemon

½ teaspoon red pepper flakes

1 teaspoon salt

1½ teaspoons freshly ground black pepper

⅓ cup extra-virgin olive oil

1. In a food processor or blender, process the spinach, basil, Parmesan cheese, walnuts, garlic, lemon juice, red pepper flakes, salt, and pepper, stopping to scrape down the sides, until it forms a fine paste.

2. With the motor running, slowly pour in the olive oil, stopping often to scrape down the sides.

Variation: **Swap the basil for one cup of sun-dried tomatoes and replace the walnuts with almonds for a completely different flavor profile.**

Per Serving: Calories: 322; Total Fat: 30g; Protein: 8g; Total Carbohydrates: 5g; Fiber: 2g; Net Carbs: 3g

Macros: Fat: 84%; Protein: 10%; Carbs: 6%

Dijon Mustard Cream Sauce

30-MINUTE / GLUTEN-FREE / ONE-POT / VEGETARIAN

This delicious cream sauce pairs well with pork, chicken, and freshly cooked vegetables. The Dijon mustard really amps up the flavor of this sauce.

SERVES

4

PREP
TIME

5

COOK
TIME

10

1 cup heavy
whipping cream

2 tablespoons
Dijon mustard

½ teaspoon red pepper
flakes (optional)

2 ounces cream cheese

1 tablespoon chopped
fresh parsley

Salt

Freshly ground
black pepper

1. In a saucepan over medium-high heat, mix together the cream, Dijon mustard, and red pepper flakes (if using) and bring to a simmer.

2. Add the cream cheese and cook for about 5 minutes, stirring often, until it reduces and slightly thickens.

3. Add the parsley and season with salt and pepper.

Variation: **Instead of Dijon mustard, use chopped sun-dried tomatoes or diced roasted red peppers.**

Per Serving: **Calories: 267; Total Fat: 27g; Protein: 3g; Total Carbohydrates: 3g; Fiber: 0g; Net Carbs: 3g**

Macros: **Fat: 90%; Protein: 5%; Carbs: 5%**

Tzatziki Sauce

30-MINUTE / GLUTEN-FREE / ONE-POT / VEGETARIAN

SERVES

PREP
TIME

This sauce pairs well with any Greek recipe, including my Simple Greek Salad (see page 37), Lamb Gyro Lettuce Boats (see page 91), and Lamb Chops with Lemon-and-Mint Asparagus (see page 92). It's bursting with fresh flavors from the lemon and dill.

½ English cucumber, peeled, seeded, and grated

¼ teaspoon salt

1 cup plain Greek yogurt

2 tablespoons chopped fresh dill

Juice of ½ lemon

5 garlic cloves, peeled

1 tablespoon extra-virgin olive oil

Freshly ground black pepper

1. Place the cucumber in a colander set over a bowl and mix it with the salt. Let sit for about 10 minutes to release any excess liquid. Place the grated cucumber into a clean kitchen towel and squeeze it to remove any remaining moisture.

2. In a food processor or blender, blend the yogurt, dill, lemon juice, garlic, and olive oil until smooth.

3. Add the cucumber to the food processor or blender with the yogurt mixture. Process for about 30 seconds, or until it reaches the consistency you prefer. Season with salt and pepper.

Make it vegan: Replace the Greek yogurt with plain coconut yogurt.

Per Serving: Calories: 104; Total Fat: 4g; Protein: 10g; Total Carbohydrates: 7g; Fiber: 1g; Net Carbs: 6g

Macros: Fat: 35%; Protein: 38%; Carbs: 27%

Cajun Seasoning

30-MINUTE / GLUTEN-FREE / ONE-POT / VEGAN

Cajun seasoning always comes in handy when you want to add a nice blackened char to any protein or a punch of flavor to your vegetables.

PREP TIME

2 teaspoons freshly ground black pepper

2 teaspoons dried oregano

2 teaspoons garlic powder

2 teaspoons onion powder

1 teaspoon dried thyme

1 teaspoon salt

1 teaspoon smoked paprika

In a jar with a lid, mix together the pepper, oregano, garlic powder, onion powder, thyme, salt, and paprika. Store at room temperature for up to 6 months.

Variation: Add some cayenne pepper if you'd prefer more heat.

Per Serving (1 teaspoon): Calories: 5; Total Fat: 0g; Protein: 0g; Total Carbohydrates: 1g; Fiber: 0g; Net Carbs: 1g;

Macros: Fat: 1%; Protein: 2%; Carbs: 97%

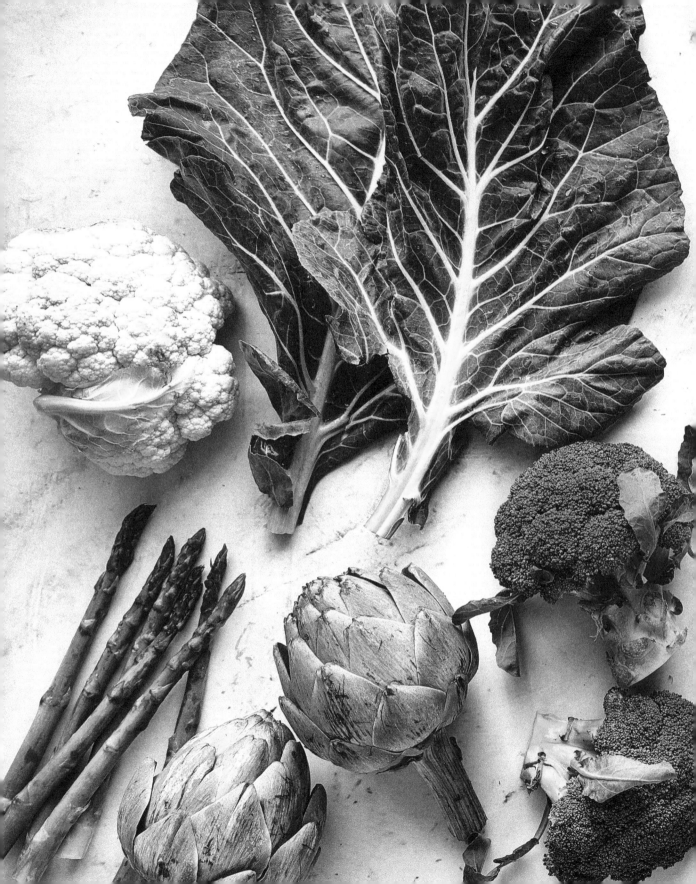

Measurement Conversions

VOLUME EQUIVALENTS (LIQUID)

US Standard	US Standard (ounces)	Metric (approx.)
2 tablespoons	1 fl. oz.	30 mL
¼ cup	2 fl. oz.	60 mL
½ cup	4 fl. oz.	120 mL
1 cup	8 fl. oz.	240 mL
1½ cups	12 fl. oz.	355 mL
2 cups or 1 pint	16 fl. oz.	475 mL
4 cups or 1 quart	32 fl. oz.	1 L
1 gallon	128 fl. oz.	4 L

OVEN TEMPERATURES

Fahrenheit (F)	Celsius (C) (approx.)
250°F	120°C
300°F	150°C
325°F	165°C
350°F	180°C
375°F	190°C
400°F	200°C
425°F	220°C
450°F	230°C

VOLUME EQUIVALENTS (DRY)

US Standard	Metric (approx.)
⅛ teaspoon	0.5 mL
¼ teaspoon	1 mL
½ teaspoon	2 mL
¾ teaspoon	4 mL
1 teaspoon	5 mL
1 tablespoon	15 mL
¼ cup	59 mL
⅓ cup	79 mL
½ cup	118 mL
⅔ cup	156 mL
¾ cup	177 mL
1 cup	235 mL
2 cups or 1 pint	475 mL
3 cups	700 mL
4 cups or 1 quart	1 L

WEIGHT EQUIVALENTS

US Standard	Metric (approx.)
½ ounce	15 g
1 ounce	30 g
2 ounces	60 g
4 ounces	115 g
8 ounces	225 g
12 ounces	340 g
16 ounces or 1 pound	455 g

Resources

General Information

Explore the following websites for more information about the low-carb diet:

- Diet Doctor: DietDoctor.com
- Ditch the Carbs: DitchTheCarbs.com
- Low Carb USA: LowCarbUSA.org
- Low-Carb Practitioners: LowCarbPractitioners.com

Apps

These smartphone applications and websites can help you track your diet and exercise:

- Carb Manager App: CarbManager.com
- My Fitness Pal: MyFitnessPal.com

Books

Bowden, Jonny. *Living Low Carb: Controlled-Carbohydrate Eating for Long-Term Weight Loss.* New York: Sterling Publishing, 2013.

Lustig, Robert H. *Fat Chance: Beating the Odds Against Sugar, Processed Food, Obesity, and Disease.* New York: Avery, 2013.

Volek, Jeff S. and Stephen D. Phinney. *The Art and Science of Low Carbohydrate Living: An Expert Guide to Making the Life-Saving Benefits of Carbohydrate Restriction Sustainable and Enjoyable.* Self-published: 2011.

References

Mayo Clinic Staff. "Low-carb diet: Can it help you lose weight?" Mayo Clinic. August 29, 2017. https://www.mayoclinic.org/healthy-lifestyle/weight-loss/in-depth /low-carb-diet/art-20045831?_ga=2.167875750.601783458.1566763412-16107742 8.1566667874.

Mayo Clinic Staff. "Paleo diet: What is it and why is it so popular?" Mayo Clinic. August 8, 2017. https://www.mayoclinic.org/healthy-lifestyle/nutrition-and -healthy-eating/in-depth/paleo-diet/art-20111182.

"Low-Carbohydrate Diets." Harvard School of Public Health. https://www.hsph .harvard.edu/nutritionsource/carbohydrates/low-carbohydrate-diets/.

Torborg, Liza. "Mayo Clinic Q and A: Make changes to stop prediabetes from developing into diabetes." Mayo Clinic. July 30, 2019. https://newsnetwork .mayoclinic.org/discussion/mayo-clinic-q-and-a-make-changes-to-stop- prediabetes-from-developing-into-diabetes/.

Recipe Label Index

Index

Acknowledgements

To Randy, my husband, best friend, and soul mate that supports me in everything I do. You are my go-to.

To Caitlyn, thank you for tolerating me as I always stand over your shoulder when you cook. Thank you for making me a mom.

To Cade, my boy, thank you for enduring my constant food and meal suggestions. You always make me smile.

To Ma, I appreciate you teaching me that a properly stocked refrigerator is made up of 90 percent condiments. I miss you!

To Dad, your love of cooking and food always inspired me. Thank you for gifting me with my passion for food.

To my siblings, I love and cherish all the priceless memories the five of us have created in the family kitchen cooking, eating, and laughing until it hurt.

To my family and friends, I sincerely appreciate your constant support and encouraging words throughout this fun journey.

To my online community, I am beyond grateful for each of you and all the amazing friendships we have developed. You inspire and motivate me on a daily basis.

About the Author

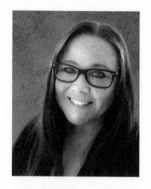

BEK DAVIS is the creator of the popular low-carb recipe and cooking tips website, Low-Carb Bek. She is a trained chef who is passionate about healthy food, and she started living a low-carb lifestyle after struggling with fad diets for decades. Having a culinary background provided her with the knowledge and creativity to assemble nutritious, low-carb meals that also taste great for herself and her family.

Bek's friends and family quickly took notice of her weight loss and asked her to share her healthy, low-carb recipes. Setting up an online presence seemed like the ideal way to share her nutritious meals with whoever needed them.

Bek lives with her husband and two teens just outside of Nashville, Tennessee. To learn more, visit her website (LowCarbBek.com) or follow her on Instagram (@LowCarbBek).